The Cancer Dancer

Healing: One Step at a Time

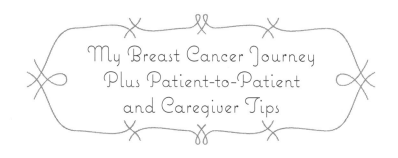

My Breast Cancer Journey
Plus Patient-to-Patient
and Caregiver Tips

Title: The Cancer Dancer
     Healing: One Step at a Time
Author: Patricia San Pedro
Cover Design: Shannon E. Coffey
Book Design: Shannon E. Coffey
Editor: Magnifico Manuscripts
Published by San Pedro Publishing
First Printing October 2011 by CreateSpace

ISBN-13: 978-0615541631   Library of Congress Number 2011916836

Printed in the United States of America

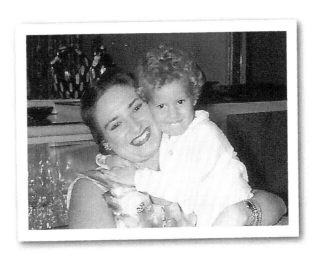

In Memory of My Beautiful Mother Daisy

Mami, you were and continue to be my inspiration.
You taught me to love unconditionally and deeply.
You may not be here physically, but your love
still flows within me. It gave me the strength
and courage to heal. Te quiero!

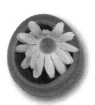

Dedications
With a profound sense of gratitude, love, and joy,
I dedicate this book to:

Tammi Leader Fuller

Tammi, you were my healing journey archangel who went to almost every single chemo treatment with me for an entire year. You baked your Bundt® cake for all the doctors and nurses. You created the angel calendar so I'd be taken care of always. You helped videotape my entire journey and log tapes. You cooked for me, loved me, and drove more miles in one year than in the lifetime of your car just to be with me. You put up with me and taught me how to be humble. You took care of me and helped me heal as we laughed our way through breast cancer. This book and my documentary would not be possible without you. Tamale, I am more grateful to you than you will ever know. I love you. Thank you.

Lydia Sacasa

Liky, I love you so much, my friend. You were my other archangel who was by my side nonstop from the moment we got the news that I had cancer. You were my rock. You joyfully accompanied me to every doctor appointment and procedure. You showered me with unconditional love, peace, and a maternal nurturing that Mami would be so touched by. You helped me heal. You cooked your deliciously delicious yummies for me. You left your family to fend for itself for an entire year so you could take care of me. I don't know how I will ever be able to express my gratitude to you properly so I will just say . . . I love you, *turuburu,* and I am forever grateful.

Annie San Roman

Annie, you took such great care of me. You were with me almost 24/7 for an entire year. We spent so many happy hours in my living room together while I chilled during chemo that it truly helped the year pass quickly. You brought joy, laughter, and delish picadillo to my life. And yes, I do know how much you love me: otherwise you would never have cleaned my kitty litter for an entire year—"mining for gold" as you called it. *Gracias, mi amiga.* Thank you.

My Family

Papi, you were there for me, as you always are. Strong. Ready to help. Full of love. You even (tried) to be positive. *Te adoro.*

Vivian, your love, kindness, compassion, and nurturing were a constant source of strength for me. I love you.

Tia *y* **Tio,** you were both there for me, always providing the love and support of family. Thank you. I love you.

Carlos and **Alex,** you are the brothers I never had. I love the way you loved me during my journey. Thank you for being there. I love you.

Table of Contents

Preface

This book is for anyone who has ever gone through a challenge that has rocked his or her world. It is for people who are healthy and need a reminder to take care of themselves and enjoy every moment of their "now."

If you have been diagnosed with breast cancer or any other disease, or love someone who has, this book is also for you. And yes, it is even for educators, the medical community, healers, insurance companies, and pharmaceutical companies, so they can get a patient's perspective of a journey they know all too well from the professional side.

No one knows what it's like to walk the breast cancer path unless she or he has walked in those same shoes. Everyone's experience is different. This is mine. I found strength, peace, and purpose in my healing journey. I have a deep sense of mission to share what I learned and help those who will walk a similar path.

In *The Cancer Dancer,* you will find very specific patient-to-patient and caregiver tips and advice that will help make the journey easier and more comfortable for you, from the day of diagnosis until the end of treatment. I used traditional healing methods but you'll also learn a little about some alternative ones that worked for me, too.

If you're inspired, I hope you'll read my story. Or, if you just want the basic information, you can skip to the back for the *Patient-to-Patient and Caregiver Tips* section.

My hope is that you unearth gems scattered throughout the pages that will help you heal better, faster, and more empowered so you can live your best new life during and after cancer.

When someone hears the words "you have cancer," it is a diagnosis for the entire family and the closest of friends. You will all travel this healing journey together. It can be a beautiful time to bond, heal, and discover new blessings in your life if you make the decision to do so.

And yes, I danced through cancer. I dance through everything in life. It's my passion. It's what makes me happy. So this wasn't any different. Of course, my dance was a very slow one at times, but it was a dance.

Whatever portion of my book you read, I hope you find healing, peace of mind, joy, and information that will help you on your own healing journey. I send you love, light, blessings, and wishes for many magical moments in your life.

Patricia San Pedro
"Positively Pat"

P.S. My lawyer friend states that nothing in this book should be taken as medical advice. You should always contact your doctor before/during/after doing anything and everything anyone might recommend in this book—no matter how logical it is!

×

Introduction: The Lesson

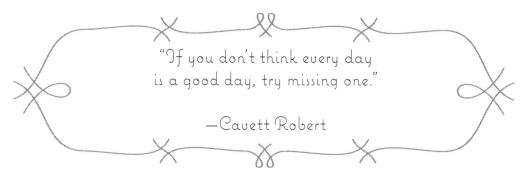

"If you don't think every day
is a good day, try missing one."

—Cavett Robert

Life is a lesson. You are the student. The universe is the teacher. You wake up one day and fall in love. Maybe you laugh a little, make love, or go to work. And then one day you wake up and life says, "You are not going to like this, but it's just what you need."

It was my birthday and I was turning 52. I received many wonderful gifts but there's only one that I will never forget—it came with a little pink ribbon. It was so small only I could see it at first. The gift card read: *You have been diagnosed with aggressive breast cancer. The recommended treatment: a double mastectomy and one year of chemotherapy.*

I thought about my mother who passed away from breast cancer 20 years ago at the age of 59. Now I had breast cancer, too. I was my mother's child; and I was alone. I didn't have a husband, boyfriend, kids, or siblings. So, what was next? What would the world bring me in all of its unpredictability? How would life hold me to its own breast?

As an eternal optimist, I quickly made a choice: my breast cancer was the pathway to a new level of heightened awareness. If God/Spirit's will was aligned with my own, I would not only survive cancer but I would thrive. I would not be a victim. My cancer would make me a better, more conscious person and I would see it as a genuine gift. I would be a guide to those facing their own disease, helping them close the gaping hole of fear. The fact that I'm writing this indicates that, at least in this case, God/Spirit and I were on the same page.

I never asked, "Why me?" I actually asked, "Why *not* me?"

Was I living in balance? Was I relaxed and not stressed? Was I eating healthy and exercising regularly? Did I live a life of peace and meditation on a regular basis? Was I living my passion? The answer was NO to all of these questions. So, maybe my cancer was the world saying, "Hey, stop and check out your life. If not now . . . *when?*"

I loved my way through cancer. I loved so hard I married the journey. You see, I was surrounded by love: friends and family who were pouring an immeasurable amount of love on me every day. This was the best memory. This was the best therapy.

My healing also came in the documentation of my passage, which was a result of my anti-silence. Why not speak to my cancer? Why not show that it didn't break me and that it actually could be a beautiful journey? I documented my healing narrative on video and on paper.

My childhood friend Maria explains:

Pat believed that documenting her journey would undoubtedly ease the path ahead for a lot of women. She became "one" with her video recorder. I never saw her without it since she was diagnosed. She videotaped every moment of her journey that she thought would be helpful to a fellow breast cancer sister. She wanted to make sure she covered all the details that no one else explained, including having safety pins available after a mastectomy; sleeping on a satin pillowcase to ease the pain after losing hair during chemotherapy; and drinking ginger or peppermint tea to alleviate nausea.

The Cancer Dancer

2008

Chapter 1: It's Cancer

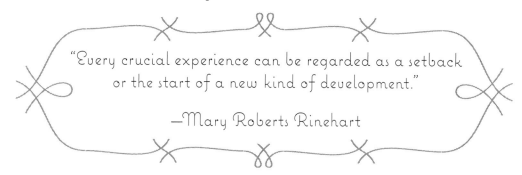

"Every crucial experience can be regarded as a setback
or the start of a new kind of development."

—Mary Roberts Rinehart

It's cancer. I know it. Last week I felt it: a bump, right on the spot where I always subconsciously checked. I had never even given myself a full breast exam which was dumb, I know. But, I always rubbed my thumb up and down on one point of my right breast. I don't know why. And now, for the first time, I felt something hard and different.

It's almost as if I've been waiting for this my whole life. When I lost my mom to breast cancer she was only 59, so I figured that the chances were pretty high that I would get it, too. But I never wasted time thinking about the possibility of getting cancer. I was not a worrier.

I was already scheduled for my annual ultrasound on April 9. My breasts were very dense and as all women who have dense breasts should do, I had an ultrasound and a mammogram every six months on a rotating basis.

I arrived for my ultrasound feeling anxious and unexpectedly uneasy. Dr. Vilma Biaggi, my radiologist, felt the lump and said, "It feels like a water cyst. Let's try to aspirate it."

Aspirating a cyst feels strange but doesn't hurt. It is just a thin needle in your breast. When water did not come out, I looked at her face.

Her jaw stiffened up as her voice changed ever so slightly. "Well, Pat, it's not water. We need to do a needle biopsy so we can properly determine what this is." At that moment a ball started to form in the pit of my stomach.

"When?" I asked.

She said, "Now. Right now. Don't worry. It won't hurt."

She pulled out another long, thin needle-contraption and went in. Strangely enough it really didn't hurt. She then said she wanted to take two samples. I wasn't liking this. As I left the room after the biopsy, Dr. Biaggi said she would call me tomorrow with the results.

I drove home feeling scared. I always try to keep positive thoughts but something about this day was different. I went about my business the rest of the day as usual. At night, before going to bed, I went to the little altar I created in my bedroom: a sweet little sacred space filled with candles, sage, precious stones, and assorted items from blessed places around the world.

I sat and I prayed; actually I pleaded. "Please don't let it be cancer. Please let my breasts be healthy." I repeated this mantra over and over again.

Then the strangest thing happened. I heard a voice. It kept interrupting my prayer request by saying, "You will use this experience to help others." Over and over as I tried to pray, I was shut down with "You will use this to help others." That's it. It's cancer. It's cancer. It's cancer.

An event that occurred 15 years ago suddenly popped into my brain. While on a business trip to Peru, I took a group of journalists to Machu Picchu in the Andes. There, as I climbed the stiff cliffs, trying to breathe, I found a tiny stone on the ground. Something compelled me to pick it up. Later that night I got violently ill. Some locals said it was because I took a stone from a sacred place.

But later on that trip, a mystical man from the Andes told me otherwise. He said "This is your stone. You will use this stone to heal yourself and others. You will make a difference on this planet."

I took the stone and brought it home. Although I had no clue what he was talking about, perhaps he knew that my world would suddenly and temporarily spin out of control.

Chapter 2: The Day of Diagnosis

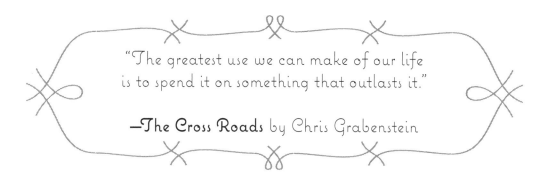

"The greatest use we can make of our life
is to spend it on something that outlasts it."

—The Cross Roads by Chris Grabenstein

Knowing that Dr. Biaggi was calling me with the results, my friend Lydia came over to be with me. She had been my friend since we were 12 years old. Already I knew I had cancer, but she didn't. I couldn't help but wonder how I would accept this news. How would she take it? How would she see me after my diagnosis?

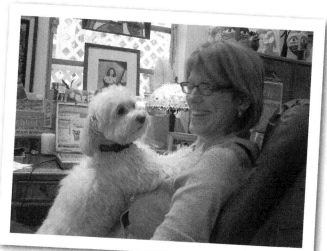

Merlot and Lydia

We prayed. Even my dog, Merlot, wanted to be a part of the action. She jumped on Lydia's lap. Then mine. Hers. Mine. Merlot sensed something.

Lydia and I went to lunch at Books & Books. When my phone rang, we looked at the number and froze. It was Dr. Biaggi. Anxiously I answered the phone and Lydia leaned in to hear the doctor say, "I'm so sorry, Pat. You have cancer."

Lydia on the day of my diagnosis:

I wanted to be with Pat when she received the results of the biopsy. I really didn't think this was cancer and I tried to reassure her. But Pat felt differently. We passed the time working in her office but after a while, I just couldn't contain myself and asked Pat to pray the rosary with me. I knew this wasn't her traditional way of praying, but I needed it and she prayed with me. I asked God for Pat's pathology report to be negative.

Typically, I am a complete worrywart; however, for some reason this time I was not worried. When the phone rang, deep inside I did not think Pat would receive negative news. I leaned in to hear the doctor say, "It's cancer" and I became numb as my heart started to pound.

With Dr. Biaggi's words, my world became silent. The air was like chalky dust and I couldn't breathe. My stomach swelled to my eyes and my brain and heart were suddenly holding each other in absolute comfort even though at times they stood in total opposition: my heart irrational, my brain logical. I wanted to divide into thousands of terrified smaller people and run away.

I heard little of what the doctor said because I was seeing and hearing the movie of my mother's life and ultimate death from breast cancer. The movie was short.

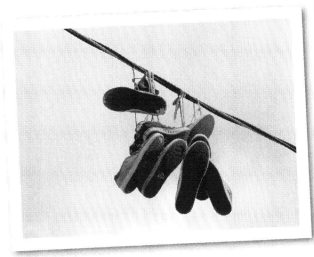

Life goes on

Dr. Biaggi suggested we meet at her office tomorrow, even though it was her day off, to make sure we understood the biopsy results. Although the tumor seemed to be encapsulated and small, the type of cancer was aggressive. Lydia and I hugged almost robotically as we tried to console each other. Neither of us could talk. We were in a daze as we walked out of the store, and I happened to look up and see shoes dangling from a phone wire where some kid had tossed them in play. I smiled and understood that the world would not stop just because I had cancer. I took a photo of the shoes to remind myself of this.

Lydia drove me home while I started calling my friends. I knew I needed to tell my dad, but I couldn't do it. Not yet. I started dialing my friends. "Tammi, I have cancer," I said as my voice broke. Lydia took the phone.

Lydia describes her reaction:

I easily could have broken down, but I didn't. I had to remain calm for her sake. As I drove Pat home, Pat started calling our friends. She had me speak to them because she couldn't get the words out. It was almost like we were actors in a play. I felt numb.

I parked in front of Pat's house and when we got out of the car, we hugged. "It's alright to cry," I told her as I began to cry. The tears we had held back so courageously finally found their way to the surface.

At six o'clock, Tammi, Mercy, Annie, Vicky, and I were sitting in Pat's living room. It was surreal. Suddenly, Pat said "Let's pop open some Champagne so we can toast my beautiful healing journey." We were shocked!

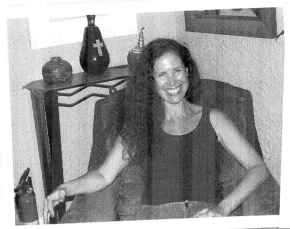

Pat four hours after diagnosis

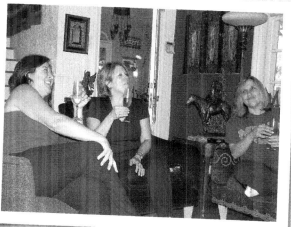

Tammi, Lydia, and Annie

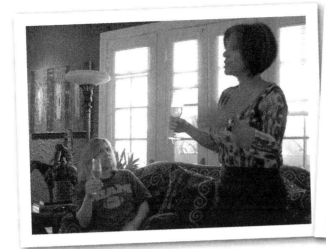

Vicky pops open Champagne

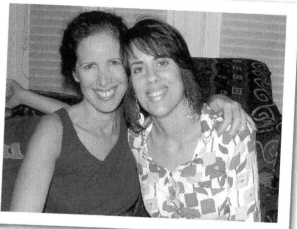

Loving hug from Mercy

She continued with a huge smile on her face, "I want to videotape the entire thing to help other women!"

What?

Pat tried to videotape here and there, but it was awkward. We didn't know what to say. Tammi picked up the camera just to humor Pat. We all thought she was in denial, but we played along.

For the rest of the night, we enjoyed each other's company. We had great conversation, watched American Idol, ate sweets, and laughed a lot. I must say that in the midst of a terrible night, we were embraced in a wonderful, loving energy where we actually had a good time. That first evening would mark the beginning of a healing journey that would not only strengthen our bond as friends, but it would confirm the mission Pat set out to accomplish seven years before when the Miami Bombshells were born. Five strangers became friends by sharing life's ups and downs and eventually writing **Dish & Tell: Life, Love, and Secrets.** *Pat created a magic carpet ride and now we were jumping onto another ride—a really scary roller coaster.*

We didn't want to leave Pat alone that night, so Tammi stayed over.

I took Merlot out for a walk under the Miami sky as Tammi prepared her bed downstairs. As I walked, I began to see the trees, the stars, even the plants, in a new way. Suddenly, I could see and feel life's movement all around me. The world was vibrant and alive, and so was I. I felt the hand of the sea breeze against my skin, and I knew that I was nature's child. Later, when I climbed into my bed, I felt a sense of complete peace, something I had never felt before. Not like that. But my brain did not yet understand what was in my heart. Was I crazy or just in denial? I had breast cancer, and yet, I felt peaceful.

Chapter 3: Calling All Angels

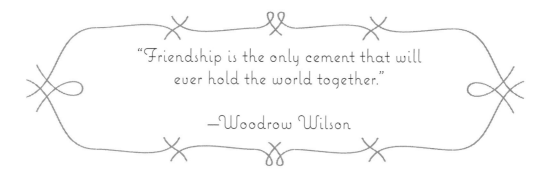

"Friendship is the only cement that will ever hold the world together."

—Woodrow Wilson

The next morning, I began thinking about my life. I never wanted children of my own and I was an only child. I married and divorced twice and my boyfriend, Mark, and I had broken up just ten days ago. Talk about timing. Long distance relationships aren't easy. He lived in Dallas and I lived in Miami. It really wasn't meant to be so we made a mutual decision to be just friends. Now I was alone. Who would take care of me?

My closest blood relative was my father, and I knew he would be a basket case once I broke the news to him. My stepmom, Vivian, was amazing but had enough on her hands taking care of my dad and her Hepatitis C. I had a loving Aunt Marta, Uncle Mario, and two cousins, Carlos and Alex, who were like my brothers. But they all had families. Everyone had a busy life.

My mind kept taking me to Mami, dying from this same thing when she was just 59. Would my story end like hers? I didn't think so. Chances for survival from cancer are much greater today. I somehow felt that my path would be different. I would not die from this. I was told I was meant to help others.

Fortunately some pretty incredible friends surrounded me; they were my sisters, my angels.

Tammi started a journal soon after my diagnosis:

In the past year, three of the closest people in my life received this horrible diagnosis. My two sisters and now Pat, my very best friend and business partner, have been diagnosed with breast cancer. Each time, it kicked me violently and deeply in the core of my gut. I wanted to throw up. The only way that breast cancer could attack me more personally is if I had it myself. I felt so helpless.

But, as I became the hand-holder and archangel to all three of these incredibly special women, I came to learn that I wasn't helpless at all. Each handled this life-challenge in their own, unique way, while my supporting role became increasingly important in this fight against the insidious enemy.

Lydia and Tammi came with me to talk to Dr. Biaggi. It wasn't an easy visit even though Dr. Biaggi was caring, compassionate, and respectful during the three hours she spent with us. She gave us the reality of my cancer.

She began, "You have infiltrating ductal carcinoma—grade three—which is a high grade. You are negative for hormone receptors. This means you are estrogen or progesterone negative— your cancer is not affected by estrogen. The good news for women with ER-negative tumors is that they derive great benefit from chemotherapy without having to take hormone therapy afterwards."

"You are positive for HER2neu, commonly referred to as HER2. This is an aggressive form of breast cancer. For women with HER2-positive breast cancers, the drug Herceptin® has been shown to dramatically reduce the risk of recurrence. It has now become standard treatment to give Herceptin along with chemotherapy after a mastectomy or lumpectomy."

"The tumor seems small at 1.7 centimeters. The good news is that you caught it early. That's very good news. But because you are HER2-positive, I'm afraid you will need to have chemo- therapy. There really is no option there. I'm sorry. But chemo is much easier these days than it used to be."

I digested all of this. What? I just couldn't believe my ears. I thought I was listening to someone else's diagnosis. As the reality sunk in, I screamed silently to myself, *Chemotherapy! She said I would need chemo. I will lose my long hair. Not Chemo! Oh my God!*

I vaguely heard her say, "You may not need a full mastectomy. A lumpectomy might be an op- tion. That's for the surgeon to determine. You should see Dr. DerHagopian. He's the best sur- geon in town. He's extremely busy, but he's a friend."

As her words swam in my head, she called her receptionist and asked to be connected to the surgeon's office. After a minute she asked me, "Can you see him Monday?" Lydia, Tammi, and I all answered at the same time.

"YES!"

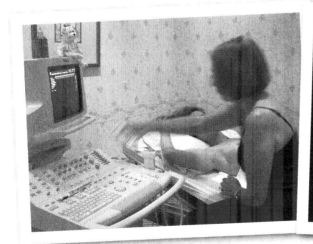
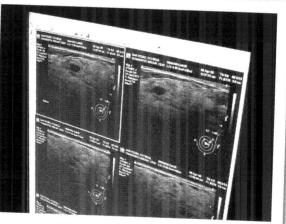

The ultrasound reveals the tumor   The Big C

I was nauseated. I continued my silent questions. *I have an option here? Should I and could I have them removed? What if the cancer returns to the other breast? This is too much to handle right now. I need to breathe.*

Dr. Biaggi took us into the ultrasound room. She wanted to take another look at me. There it was front and center. It wasn't a mistake.

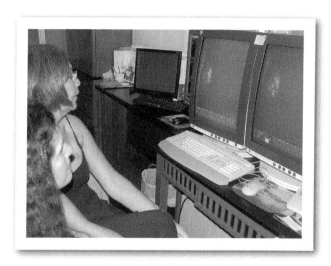

Looking at the results

Chapter 4: Write It All Down:
The Good, The Bad, and the Yucky

"People do not 'have' diseases, which are really descriptive mechanisms created by contemporary medicine. People have stories, and the stories are narratives of their lives, their relationships, and the way they experience an illness."

—Arthur Kleinman

I spent the rest of the day educating myself on breast cancer. Tammi and I met with a friend, Sally Bogert, who worked in the breast cancer industry. She provided us with a lot of information that prepared us for the surgeon's visit on Monday.

Infiltrating Ductal Carcinoma (IDC) means atypical cells mutate as they grow. They gather in the ducts in the breast. The cells break through the duct wall and move into the surrounding tissue. This is when the cancer crosses the line from Ductal Carcinoma In Situ (DCIS) to IDC.

Tumor grade is a method of classifying cancer cells with reference to how abnormal they look under a microscope and how quickly the tumor is likely to grow and spread. Grades range from 1 to 4 where 1 is considered the least aggressive. I had Grade 3.

She also said I wouldn't know what stage my cancer was until I had the surgery. But as of right now, from the pathology report, I was Stage 1. That was good.

By late afternoon, I was exhausted. I decided that I was going to make this weekend all about me. I went to a concert and spent time with my girlfriends. I pampered myself. I took a few pictures and videos of me with my hair, knowing that it might be just a memory in the near future.

I wanted to remember what I really looked like.

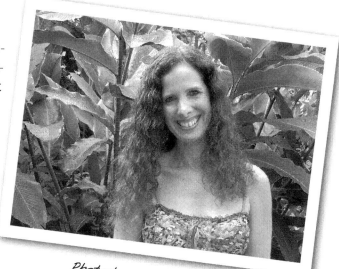

Photo to remember my hair

I began to clear the clutter from my house so I would have a healthy, flowing, and happy atmosphere in which to heal. I began to journal about my process. I saw journaling as a way to reflect on my healing. In a way, my journal would capture the memory of my cancer and the hope of a cancer-free future. It would be a method of conversation with myself. I would gather information, comfort, and motivate myself and others, and begin the journey of healing through expression. There would be no silence in sickness. I wrote for my life and the lives of others.

Pat's Journal: April 12, 2008

I was diagnosed two days ago. I think that this is going to be a process. I'm praying and meditating that it's all going to be fine. I have an amazing support system behind me with my wonderful and amazing girlfriends. I'm scared but at the same time I am at peace. I'm keeping this written journal and a videotaped diary of my journey to raise awareness and stress the importance of early detection. I also want other women to see that I'm not freaking out. I'm okay. Of course, I have waves of emotion. I am human. But I must trust, have faith, and be positive.

Pat's Journal: April 14, 2008

I'm going to see the surgeon for the first time today. This visit will change my life forever. I know it will be tough and scary, but I'm praying that I'll keep my peace of mind and that everyone around me will remain positive. Author Robin Sharma wrote, "Those of us who are seekers, who want to better ourselves, will always go through HUGE obstacles in our lives, and how we face them determines how we come out on the other side." This will definitely be a healing journey. And waiting on the other side of this is going to be beauty and healing for others.

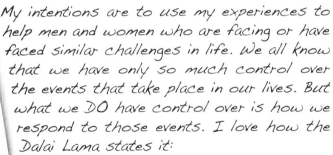

My intentions are to use my experiences to help men and women who are facing or have faced similar challenges in life. We all know that we have only so much control over the events that take place in our lives. But what we DO have control over is how we respond to those events. I love how the Dalai Lama states it:
"Pain is inevitable. Suffering is optional."

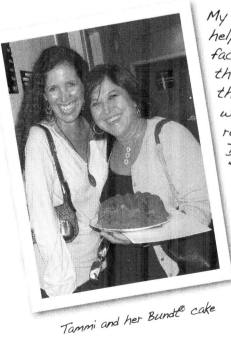

Tammi and her Bundt® cake

Tammi baked a Bundt cake. "You want the staff happy," she said and smiled. So off I went with my archangels Lydia and Tammi and Tam's spongy cake.

Robert P. DerHagopian, MD, FACS, surgical oncologist, had more than 40 years of experience in his field. He was a winner of both the **Patients' Choice Award** and **One of America's Top Doctors Award**. His stellar reputation spanned the planet. He was compassionate and kind. Dr. D took his time examining my breasts and calmly described the diagnosis in great detail.

"I'm still not sure whether a lumpectomy or mastectomy is needed—"

I quickly interrupted. "My breasts are attached to me; I'm not attached to them. Take them both off!"

He smiled and explained, "There are three tests to help us determine the full depth of the diagnosis: an MRI of the breasts, a PET scan, and the BRCA Gene Test since you have a history of breast cancer in your family. The tumor is only 1.7 centimeters which is good news. Of course, we won't know how to proceed until all the tests are run and you have your surgery." He wasn't alarming when he spoke and he made it seem like it was all okay. He was a doll.

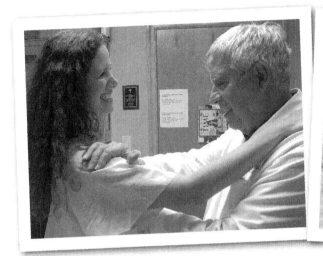 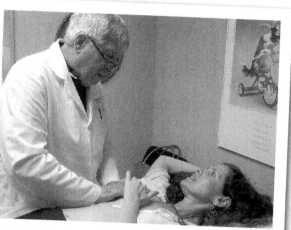

Dr. DerHagopian examines me   Dr. DerHagopian feels the tumor

Pat's Journal: April 16, 2008

Today I am going for my MRI and BRCA Genetic Test. Vicky will take me to both. I am nervous since I don't know what to expect. I do know that the MRI gives detailed images of my breasts which will allow the doctors to better evaluate the presence of cancer. I am surrounded by angels, love, light, and healing. I might have cancer, but I feel so blessed. But why did I get this?

"YOU HAVE CANCER SO YOU CAN HEAL YOURSELF AND OTHERS, TO RECEIVE LOVE IN WAYS THAT YOU NEVER HAVE BEFORE, AND TO FULLY UNDERSTAND THAT YOU ARE LOVED!"

Wow! I don't think I can write this down fast enough! I think I'm experiencing Automatic Writing. It is a type of channeling where God or Spirit flows through you to communicate, guide, and create the words. I would get answers to my questions. Very cool! Of *course, I'm skeptical. What if it's really me answering my own questions? I guess it doesn't matter. If the answers help me, then hurray!*

Let the light of God and all my beautiful angels descend now upon me and in my life as I begin this healing process and enter into my healing journey. I am grateful, I am whole, and I am at peace.

Upon arriving at Baptist Outpatient Services center, Vicky and I were greeted by warm and caring personnel that made such a difference. Pablo was the nurse assistant that would walk me through the process. I was so thankful for his help. As we waited, I started to stretch. I pulled my arms to the side . . . up . . . down . . . and moved my head around. I wanted to be as relaxed and as flexible as possible for this process that would put me into a strange position for a long time.

"Please change into the robe in the dressing room," Pablo said.

He then walked me to the MRI room. There was a glass booth that looked like control central with several people behind it. The MRI machine was a large cylinder-shaped tube. Pablo explained, "The machine will move up and down your body to take images of your breasts. It is critical that you stay totally still throughout the process."

Easier said than done. Pablo positioned me face down and strapped me into the white bed. He placed my hands along the sides of the table and my breasts hung freely into plastic openings. Why isn't anything cushioned? I wondered.

I learned that the best way to stay still was to make sure I was completely comfortable before starting and that I was relaxed and my muscles were not tense.

Make sure you tell the technologist if something is uncomfortable before you start. The more comfortable you are (within limits), the best chance you have to get it over with quickly. Even a tiny movement will make them have to start all over again.

Pablo's final instructions were a warning. "You will hear very loud noises."

He wasn't kidding. There were VERY LOUD NOISES!

The MRI went well. It took about 30 minutes. I meditated myself away, envisioning the thunderous noise to be Indian drums and chants. All healing. The mind was very powerful.

From there we went for the blood test for the genetic testing. That didn't go so well. My veins were tiny. They rolled. Imploded. Hid. It took five tries and still nothing. Vicky looked at me. I looked at her at which point I said "I'm outta here." We walked out and made an appointment for another day. I would drink gallons of water the night before next time to pump up my veins. I went back a week later. This time it worked. Now it would take about two to three weeks to get the results.

Pat's Journal: April 17, 2008

Will I be okay?

"YES! YES! THE PROCESS WILL BE EASIER THAN YOU EXPECT. GIFTS ARE COMING! MANY BLESSINGS ARE HEADED YOUR WAY. YOU WILL ENCOUNTER LIFE'S CHANGES, EXPERIENCE DIFFERENT TRANSITIONS, PARTAKE IN JOURNEYS UNKNOWN AND FACE INCREDIBLE CHALLENGES. NO MATTER IF THEY'RE GREAT OR SMALL, LET GO AND RELEASE! GOT IT?"

Yes, I got it. I am grateful, I am healing, and I am whole. Tomorrow I will get a full-body PET Scan to see if the cancer has spread. I know in the deepest part of my soul that it's going to be okay, but a little confirmation would really be nice.

The Cancer Dancer

Chapter 5: Faith
(and a PET Scan)

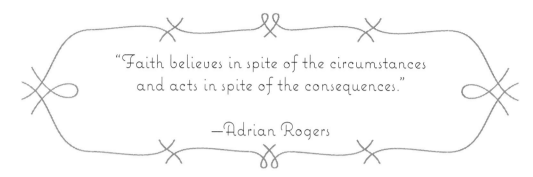

*"Faith believes in spite of the circumstances
and acts in spite of the consequences."*

—Adrian Rogers

Lydia picked me up to take me to my PET Scan at Baptist Hospital. I was a little nervous since I never had a procedure done like this before. But the scan would tell me whether I had cancer anywhere else in my body.

We were taken into a small room where they gave me an intravenous injection of radioactive glucose. This time the technician found my vein easily. They had me lay down and sent Lydia to the waiting room. I stared at the ceiling and tried to relax. It was all so weird: waiting to hear whether your cancer was even worse than what it already was. The staff wouldn't even let me read a book as I needed to be perfectly still. I was told to do nothing. I needed complete silence and quiet. So I used the time to meditate about health and healing.

After about an hour, the technician came to get me. We went into the PET Scan room and once again they laid me on a cool table. This time I was face up with my hands above my head. Compared to an MRI, the machine was a bigger cylinder tube and the room seemed a bit larger. There was a control room but it was larger also. The table where I was to lay down would move up and down through the cylinder scanner. I brought with me one of my favorite music CDs, *Sky Spirit*. It was Indian flute music and would send me to a transient state, a beautiful place. I asked the technician, "Can you play this for me while I am having the scan?"

He smiled and said, "Of course."

Once inside the tube, I was still. This time as I listened to the loud noises and associated them with Native American chants, I made up chants in my head to go with the beat of the noises.

"I am healed. I am healthy. Yes I am. I am healed. I am healthy. Yes I am." I listened to the music's slight hum. I closed my eyes and looked through the slit of my closed eyelids. I envisioned Divine Light coming from God/Spirit to heal me. I saw the warmth of the world hover over me and hold me in the light. It was life spreading its arms to touch my hand and it was life whispering in my ear, "You are healthy. You are healing."

Lydia tells the story while I was inside the Pet Scan area:
While accompanying Pat on one of her many doctor's appointments, I found that during difficult times laughter is still the best medicine.

It started as just another appointment for another test. However, this afternoon turned out to be a much longer one than we expected. Pat had to undergo a PET Scan to see if the cancer had spread to other parts of her body. We were at Baptist Hospital going through the registration process, getting the paperwork done quickly, and then heading to the imaging waiting area.

Once there, we were led to another waiting room just outside the "Active Radiation" area where Pat would have her test done. The nurse asked me to leave as Pat was supposed to stay very still during this process. They turned the lights off in her room and I left. I was getting anxious, and was happy to leave since I did not want my anxiety to rub off on Pat. Being the shopaholic that I am, I went to the gift shop and mulled around.

I headed back to the small waiting room confident that I still had plenty of time left to find Pat before they took her in. But when I arrived, she was gone. Maybe I went to the wrong place or took a wrong turn. Everything was gray and the hospital walls started to look the same to me. I walked around for a few minutes, and then I heard it. I stood still to make sure that I wasn't going crazy. I was hearing Native American flutes; how was that possible in the hospital?

I followed the music and was led to large double doors where a sign stopped me in my tracks: "Prohibited. Active Radiation."

I put my ear to the door and listened. It WAS Native American flutes. I wasn't going crazy. I started to laugh. The people around me stared as they must have thought I had suddenly flipped. However, I had found my friend. I couldn't see her, but I knew that behind those doors was Pat, serene and calm, having her test as she listened and floated away to her favorite music which connected her to God, Mother Earth, the universe, and all her angels.

Chapter 6: I Guess I'm Not Dreaming

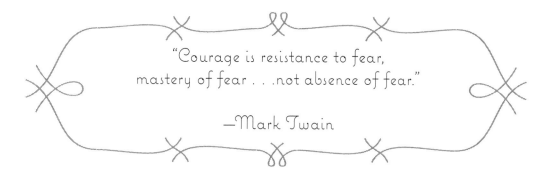

"Courage is resistance to fear, mastery of fear . . .not absence of fear."

—Mark Twain

I went to see a medical oncologist *before* my mastectomy. Most surgeons tell you to wait until the surgery is over before you see an oncologist. However, I wanted to choose my medical oncologist and get input before I had my surgery. I followed my friend Sally's advice of finding the right one before my surgery.

"You might need to see two or three oncologists before finding the one you feel comfortable with. A medical oncologist will give you valuable information."

I saw one medical oncologist who I liked, but she wasn't the one. The moment I met Dr. Stefan Glück, my search was over. This man was compassionate, nurturing, and a leader in his field.

Dr. Stefan Glück, MD, FRCP(C), PhD, was a professor of medicine at the University of Miami, my alma mater. He was also Associate Division Chief for Clinical Affairs, Division of Hematology/Oncology, and Clinical Director at the Braman Family Breast Cancer Institute at the University of Miami's Sylvester Comprehensive Cancer Center. He was internationally known for his work on breast cancer, head and neck cancer, and bone marrow transplants.

Lydia accompanied me on this first visit to Dr. Glück's office. She took notes for me as my head began to spin with the abundance of information. He gave us the statistics and the information on the drugs I would need. He answered all of my questions.

"Should I get a mastectomy or a lumpectomy?"

He gave us tons of numbers that had me leaning towards a mastectomy.

"How long until my hair falls out?"

He said usually about ten days after the first chemo treatment.

"How quickly should I start my chemotherapy?"

"I don't think you should delay chemo as you are Her2-positive. About three weeks after your surgery," he calmly replied.

"Should I drink lots of water before or after my chemo? Will I get an allergic reaction to the treatments?"

He patiently explained, "Yes. Lots of water during and after chemo to flush it out of your body. We give you pre-meds to avoid allergic reactions."

"How sick should I expect to get? How many treatments do I need?"

He gave me his full attention. "You will need seventeen sessions of chemo every three weeks for one year."

I put my complete trust in this man. He was yet another healing angel placed in my path.

I was somewhat concerned as I remembered my mom, Daisy, going through her chemo treatments 20 years earlier. They weren't fun. She would get really, really sick. She would throw up. She would be in pain. I had blocked many of these memories from my mind; I just remember her being very ill. But once again, I knew current treatments were different. I would get through this, I would have fun in the process, and I would help others with what I would learn.

Dr. Glück's wonderful nurse, Jennifer Herrera Perdigon, asked me when I would like to have my chemo.

Lydia recounted this:

She told Pat she could schedule her every third week on a Thursday or Friday. They usually try and schedule patients for those days so they can have a recovery period during the weekend and go back to work on Monday. Pat looked at her and said, "Why in the world would I do that?" Jennifer looked at Pat like she was crazy. Pat smiled and said, "I wanna have fun on the weekends honey—you schedule me for Monday or Tuesday." We all cracked up. Dr. Glück laughed as he said, "Nobody in my thirty years of medicine has ever said that." We actually had a great time at the doctor's office.

Another wonderful angel from Dr. Glück's office gave us a tour of CTU (the unit where you get chemo). It was a good idea to see this place before the actual first day of treatment.

I was a bit nervous as we walked into this huge room filled with cubicles. There were many people receiving chemo and nurses all around them. The atmosphere however was peaceful and the nurses were warm and friendly.

Then someone called my name. "Patty!"

Was I hearing things? I heard it again. "Patricia!"

I looked around to find a man. He looked vaguely familiar but I couldn't place him.

"It's Max!" he said.

"Max?" I didn't get it.

Then he said, "It's Orfirio."

"Oh my God!"

Orfirio and I had grown up together. We were friends during high school, college, and beyond and I hadn't seen him in over 20 years. We hugged.

"I am a chemo nurse in this unit."

I started to cry. His eyes filled with tears as did Lydia's. He was another angel God had placed onto my healing journey. This time it was my chemo nurse. This was just unbelievable.

As I looked at him, I saw that it was really him—just a bit heavier (sorry) and a lot grayer. His huge, bright eyes and warm laughter were the same. He was known to me as Orfirio but at the hospital they called him Max.

I made a note to myself to request him as my chemo nurse. We left feeling uplifted, happy, and hopeful.

I had my surgeon, my chemo nurse, and my oncologist. Now I needed a plastic surgeon to give me the full C-cup I had always wanted. I never wanted it this way, but this was reality. I am going to lose my breasts to cancer. There was nothing left to do but pray and write about it.

Pat's Journal: April 18, 2008

Maybe it's finally hitting me? I woke up sad today. I guess more than I realized. Maybe I just needed to exhale a bit, but it's okay. I want to go dancing this weekend. I want to have fun! I spent wonderful quality time with Mercy and it felt good. Just like we learned in the Andes from shamans, we performed a beautiful healing ceremony. This meant so much to me.

Tammi and Lydia haven't left my side since the diagnosis. I do not know what I would do without them. They have left their families to fend for themselves and have been glued to me ever since. Lydia is even asking La Luna (the moon) to heal me. Praying to the moon is so "me", not Lydia. I love it!

Annie and Mercy have also made themselves available to me nonstop. Maria is in New York. I won't tell her until she returns.

Now I'm waiting for the results of my PET Scan. This waiting is making us all a little bit crazy. Sure cancer is present, but I feel that it's only in my right breast. Somehow, I just know it! The questions now are: What's taking so long? When will the doctor call?

I'm sitting around twiddling my thumbs, waiting for this news that I desperately need to share with my dad. I want to give him the full picture. I don't want to put him through this wait-and-see and the anxiety that I'm experiencing.

Tammi has a date tonight. She's so excited. This will be the first date that she's been on since her last breakup. I hope she has fun, although I know she's on pins and needles waiting for my scan results. Lydia is going to a concert. She, too, is nervous as hell, but trying to hide it from me. I can see right through her. Annie is a wreck too! I know because she's being unusually up and chirpy. That means she's really worried.

I'm going to Vicky's tonight. We're going to drink champagne with friends and just try to forget about the scan. I'll worry about the call when I get it.

I remember that night so well. We were on our second glass of Champagne when my cell phone rang.

"It's Dr. D," I nervously told everyone. I fumbled for my journal to take notes. I always took notes.

Dr. D began speaking. "Pat, it's good news. The PET Scan is clean. You have multi-focal disease in more than one area of the breast but no where else. You might be a better candidate for a mastectomy, but a lumpectomy is still an option. Even though it's Her2neu-positive, this is the best news possible!"

I turned to my friends and smiled a half-smile. I put the cell on speaker so they could all hear what he had to say. He talked about the pros and cons of lumpectomy versus mastectomy: the failure rate was eight percent over ten years which means that 92 percent of women who choose to have a lumpectomy will have no recurrence in ten years. But eight percent will have either a new cancer or a recurrence. He also said that the disadvantage with going the lumpectomy route is that I would need radiation in addition to the chemo. But if I got a mastectomy, I would need only chemo. Dr. D said that the need for chemo is a biological need and is independent of the operation being done.

I hung up the phone, numb at first, and then we all hugged. I spoke to myself. *Thank you God. I have cancer, but I am thrilled. It has not spread.*

My happiness ran through me like a quick shock. I looked at all my friends sitting there and my heart was joyful and tight with love. It was as if the moment took me into its own breasts and I could feel the warmth of total and complete love. I hadn't digested the pros and cons yet of the surgery, but tonight was for celebrating.

When I got home, Annie was waiting with a bottle of red wine. We walked outside, holding hands, and under the full moon we prayed. Annie cried and cried and just kept kissing my cheeks over and over again. I cried, too.

I thought, *This cancer is bearing many gifts. So many people love me very much. I am truly blessed. Who knew that cancer wasn't sour? For me it's brought sweetness, kindness, and compassion. Who knew?*

Pat's Journal: April 19, 2008

I have never been more convinced that part of my healing encompasses healing others, including my dad. For many, I will be a conduit for healing. It is the shamanic way. I am blessed to have been chosen. I get confirmation of that ten times a day. I'll just wait and tell Papi and Vivian tomorrow. Then Tia y Tio, my wonderful Aunt Marta and Uncle Mario.

Pat's Journal: April 20, 2008

I'm looking forward to Unity on the Bay service today. I love this place. The energy is amazing and Rev. Chris Jackson's sermons truly bring such clarity to my life. I need the strength to tell Papi about my cancer. I will tell him tonight. I need to get this off my chest. Literally! How do I tell him?

"QUIETLY, GENTLY, LOVINGLY, CALMLY. WHEN YOU GIVE HIM ALL OF THE DETAILS, HE WILL UNDERSTAND. WHEN YOU ARE READY, GRADUALLY START EXPLAINING WITH A CYST. THEN 'CANCER,' BUT INCLUDE THAT IT IS 100% CURABLE. THAT IT'S JUST IN THE BREASTS, NOWHERE ELSE. BEAUTY WILL COME FROM THIS. AT UNITY, YOU WILL FIND A WAY. CAREFULLY LISTEN TO THE WORDS. THEY WILL HELP AND GUIDE YOU. BE THE LIGHT!"

Pat's Journal: April 21, 2008

Papi had a bad cold last night. Guess I'm not supposed to tell him yet.

Pat's Journal: April 22, 2008

I am healthy, whole, and complete. Now—today!

This is a good time for me to place things into perspective. I need to keep only positive people and good thoughts around me. I'll start by releasing feelings of betrayal, and then I'll release all hurt and resentment. With this release I am free! I am a spirit. I am whole. I am good—and I love me!

Oh wow, I just got the call from the plastic surgeon's office. Dr. Marshall had a cancellation and could see me in half an hour. Okay, I'll be there. I'll throw on some clothes and call Lydia.

Chapter 7: No Breasts – New Breasts

> "Scars signify an ongoing battle and that all is not lost.
> As befits one of nature's great triumphs, scar tissue is
> a magical substance, a physiological and psychological
> mortar that holds flesh and spirit together when a
> difficult world threatens to tear both apart."
>
> —Armando Favazza

Lydia met me at Dr. Dierdre Marshall's office. I still had not made a decision on whether or not I wanted to have a lumpectomy or a bilateral mastectomy, though I was leaning toward the mastectomy.

Dr. Marshall informed me that by removing both breasts, the additional threats of more cancer would be removed. She continued, "I've never heard a patient say 'I wish I hadn't had a mastectomy.'"

My options were to get implants or have a flap procedure. The benefit of a flap is that your breasts would be rebuilt with your own fat. The negative is that it is major, major surgery and very traumatic to the body. I didn't like that option so I decided on the less traumatic: implants.

The next step was to take pictures of my breasts. Dr. Marshall's photographer, Joe, made me feel as comfortable as he could. I disrobed, took off my bra, and closed my eyes as he took pictures of my breasts. It was quick and I tried not to think about how my new breasts would look.

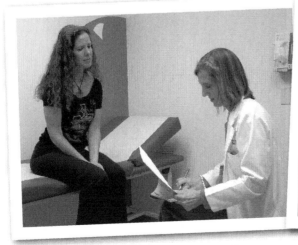

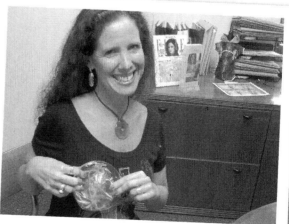

Dr. Marshall explains the options   Time to pick my cup size

From there we went to see Erica to give me a tour of Dr. Marshall's patients—all in different stages of reconstruction. I thought the reconstruction would look unbearable and painful—bruised breast and deformed shapes—but there wasn't any of that. I started to feel comforted by the realness of it all.

Afterward, I went cup-size shopping. Did I want a B-cup like I had, or should I go for the gusto and decide on a C-cup? It took me less than a nanosecond to decide. I chose the full C. I would be slightly voluptuous and curvy. I would have—*drum roll please!*—cleavage! The plan was for Dr. Marshall to do an immediate reconstruction.

Dr. D would do the mastectomy and then Dr. Marshall would come into the operating room to place the expanders in me. Every few weeks I would return to Dr. Marshall's office to be expanded. They would inject saline into the expanders and pump to expand my skin gradually. The whole process would take about six months, which was okay with me. I was in no hurry.

Pat's Journal: April 23, 2008

I feel whole. I feel so loved. I am healed. But I don't want chemo! I will be positive. My cells are all healthy. I will pray the cancer away.

We're all capable of choosing how we feel and how we deal with circumstances. If I freak out, how will that help me? So I am choosing to remain calm and positive, even when I'm all alone and no one else is around, I'm fine, really. I saw the plastic surgeon yesterday and loved her. She will be right behind the surgical oncologist on surgery day, beginning to rebuild the new breasts that will one day be mine.

Chapter 8: Energy Medicine, Feeding Faith

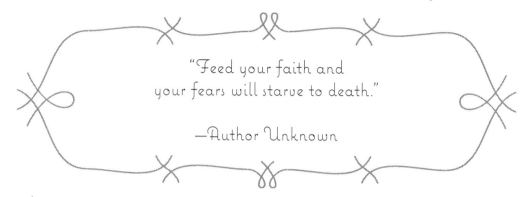

"Feed your faith and
your fears will starve to death."

—Author Unknown

As soon as I was diagnosed, I called Dr. Claudia Edwards, a dear friend, psychologist, and shamanic healer. I wanted every type of healing I could get to help me on my journey. I would use the traditional form of healing (surgery and chemotherapy) but on a parallel course, I wanted to take advantage of energy medicine, too. Claudia and I studied energy medicine together in Peru, along with Mercy. Our mentor was Dr. Alberto Villoldo from **The Four Winds Shamanic Organization.** We had learned about this first-hand when we visited and learned from the shamans in the Amazon Jungle and the Andes in Peru. A shaman works with the energies all around us. It is an ancient healing practice that works with the energy fields that surround the body. At one point in my life I would have totally rolled my eyes at this weird stuff. But not anymore.

There are many different practices of energy medicine and this field is referred to by different names including Electromagnetic Energy Field, Chi, or Luminous Energy Field. The energy field is a template for physical, emotional, and stress-related problems, and connects to the physical body through the seven chakras (energy centers of our body). The goal of all forms of energy medicine is to restore the healthy flow of the energy field, healing by restoring homeostasis to the body.

Claudia explains this best:

Shamanic energy medicine in the tradition of the Peruvian Incas is both a spiritual and healing practice based in the belief that the universe is a web of energy and spirit that sustains all life. Shamans are masters at communicating with the spirit of everything in nature, and navigating through these energy fields to effect change. By learning how to use your breath, emotions, and intentions, both the shaman and client can make interventions in the energy field that surrounds the body, as well as the energy fields that exists between people (known as relationships), and between people and their environment. Bringing ourselves into balance with the natural world around us creates shifts in the energy field that surrounds the physical body influencing health and well-being.

Shamanism is not a religion and is not in conflict with any religion. There is a spiritual component of shamanism which is based on the principles of impeccability, integrity, sustainability, and care-taking for the earth and all of its inhabitants.

As soon as Claudia heard of my cancer, she sent me an email:

Pat,

Today, I will put a healing stone in my mesa (my medicine bag) for you, and will ask Spirit to wrap her coils of light around you leaving a small opening at your crown chakra to let the light of spirit in. You will be guided and protected on this healing journey. If you send me the names of your doctors, I will also wrap them in the light with the intention that they will be called to their most skilled selves and their highest potential. If you need surgery, I always like to wrap the operating room as well, so keep me up-to-date.

In the meantime, keep working as sisters; it is more powerful when we work together, so even if you can't all be in the same physical place, hold space together to heal. Remember that the ultimate power of the universe is love, and the greatest power of the feminine is community; so do not underestimate the power that exponentially grows when sisters sit together in love with a common purpose. We cannot have fear here, so if you can't keep it out of your own field, then just step out of the healing field until you regain positive focus.

Finally, Pat, you can greet your tumor as a worthy opponent and begin a dialogue with it. Writing exercises are good ways to do this. Here is a poem that may also help. It has withstood the test of time.

"The Guest House"

This being human is a guest house.
Every morning a new arrival.

A joy, a depression, a meanness,
some momentary awareness comes
as an unexpected visitor.

Welcome and entertain them all!
Even if they're a crowd of sorrows,
who violently sweep your house
empty of its furniture,
still, treat each guest honorably.
He may be clearing you out
for some new delight.

The dark thought, the shame, the malice,
meet them at the door laughing,
and invite them in.

Be grateful for whoever comes,
because each has been sent
as a guide from beyond.

~

Rumi

I will be happy to support you on this journey, dear sister. Please let me know how I can help you even further.

Love and light to you all,
Claudia

Susan Wittig Albert wrote, "Storytelling is healing. As we reveal ourselves in story, we become aware of the continuing core of our lives under the fragmented surface of our experience."

My energy medicine was part of my healing story and even permeated throughout my written and videotaped journals. It was as if my journals became the energy that would save me. I wrote and wrote, videotaped and videotaped, and filled it all with beautiful, bright, shining, divine light and healing. This was the energy surrounding my healing journey.

Tammi, Mercy, Maria, and Vicky came with me to a healing ceremony led by Claudia. So did Stefanie, who had been my next-door neighbor for years. She's a special person who works with children and therapy dolphins. Kathi also joined us. She's the producer of our Bombshell Musical, but our connection had gone to friendship in a heartbeat.

Pat's Journal: April 25, 2008

I am feeling such incredible balance and harmony and feeling so at one with God/Spirit. Claudia Edwards was great yesterday. All my angels showed up for her ceremony, even though many did not understand any of it.

During this energy healing ritual, I literally blew my cancer into a stone that Mercy had brought from Machu Picchu. I could actually feel the unhealthy cells leaving my body and going right into the stone that we had found together in Peru. The same place where 15 years earlier, I found the stone that the medicine man said would one day be used to heal others and myself. It sent an eerie chill down my spine, but in a good way.

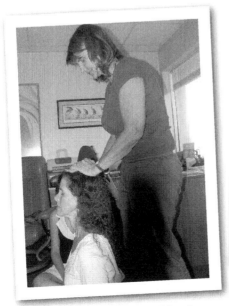

Energy healing with Claudia

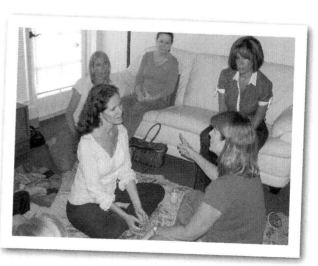

My friends watch and learn

When I got home I made a mandala in my backyard. A mandala is a visual form of Hindu prayer. I picked up sticks, twigs, flowers—anything I wanted—and created a beautiful healing circle in thoughtful prayer. My intent was healing. Tibetan Buddhists created intricate sand mandalas that sometimes took days to complete. I buried the stone in the center. I put all my cancer in the stone, through my intent, so the earth (the Pachamama) would mulch it and take it away from me. Like I said before, this would have been very crazy talk in years past, but now I was a believer.

After the intensity at Claudia's, my angels took me belly dancing at the Wellness Community Center. Dancing and moving the body is just as healing as anything else. We had a blast! Once again, I realized that laughter is the best medicine.

Over the weekend I went to see a spiritual teacher named Patrick Connor. A friend invited me to a gathering of spiritually-seeking people. Since healing was my main mission, I spent the weekend praying with Patrick and 20 strangers who came together to learn and grow. And it was here where I finally broke down. I prayed until I really began to see myself in the present.

I had cancer. I was going to lose my breasts. Would I survive? I sobbed like a baby. Out loud. I felt my mother's death. I felt my fear. And then, as the tears kept flowing, I released it. It was over. I felt as if I had been cleansed. It was exhausting but totally empowering at the same time. I was almost ready for the doctors to reconstruct my body. Patrick gave me an affirmation to recite, and he told me to say it 400 times a day.

Daily Affirmation

I am beautiful and perfect exactly as I am.
I AM that I AM.

There is only God. There is only Love.
I see all beings as beautiful and perfect.
There is no such thing as illness or death.
And no such thing as cancer.
I am no longer subject to these ideas.
There is nothing outside of me to fear.
I am the energy of Love itself.
I am an eternal and infinite being.

Patrick also instructed, "Visualize your body filled with light. Do the meditation we did with the ball of golden white light going up the back of the spine and down the front. Do that each day."

And I did do it. Every day. I still do it every day. I believe that my winning combination to wellness is daily affirmations, meditation, and prayer; faith; the love of my family and friends; laughter; love; and a positive attitude.

Pat's Journal: April 26, 2008

I went for a second ultrasound, just to see what was up. It showed that the two tumors had grown legs. Crap! I thought I might be able to reduce them or zap them away with prayer, but it didn't work. This baby really is aggressive. Surgery is scheduled for May 31 but Dr. D doesn't want to wait. I want this out of me. Bilateral mastectomy is my decision. I know that this is the right choice, but I still think it's weird to take both breasts without having to, especially since I am single. Who will want to be with me? Who really cares right now? I have a lot of life yet to live.

Right now I want and need peace of mind! So, if there's no breast tissue left, the breast cancer can't grow, right?

I went dancing tonight with Tammi and Annie. It's official: this is now a part of my healing process and boy, do I love to dance. I'm going to the Keys this weekend. Next weekend is my surgery. I need to be carefree without having to go to doctor appointments or visits with specialists.

Chapter 9: True Confessions

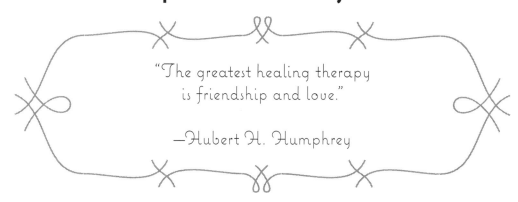

"The greatest healing therapy is friendship and love."

—Hubert H. Humphrey

Back in 2005 when my girlfriends and I wrote **Dish & Tell,** we also created a back-to-nature, women-only weekend retreat called Camp Bombshell. It was an escape . . . a time for women across the country to reconnect with themselves by leaving their men, stress, kids and make-up at home and taking a time-out for themselves. We would do yoga, dance, sing by the campfire, and jump off zip-lines. The retreats were fun and healing at the same time. A beautiful bond developed between many of the women who became regular campers. We had a total of 13 camps over the past three years. The last one happened right before my mastectomy.

Pat's Journal: May 1, 2008

Vicky drove me to Camp. I didn't go early as I usually do to help set up. I had a lot on my mind and hadn't decided whether or not I was even going. Finally, Vicky said she'd drive me. We arrived at Camp Bombshell late in the day. The peace I felt for the past three weeks had quickly melted away. I was starting to crash. When I arrived at camp, I found a note on my bunk written by my archangel Tammi:

"Welcome my friend . . . to the place where you belong right now. Communing with nature and people who really, truly, love you from the inside out. Take it in. Receive it all with open arms.

Let the healing begin,
xoxoxox Tammi

I stepped out onto the beautiful campgrounds and saw campers I hadn't seen since the year before. Anne Sussman from New Jersey, one of the girls I'd grown closest to, ran up to me and grabbed me and whisked me away to chat by the lake. It was so good to see her but I had an awful feeling in the pit of my stomach that wouldn't let me relax.

Anne quickly brought me up to speed on her life and then proceeded to talk for half an hour about a friend of hers who was diagnosed with breast cancer. I was speechless. I couldn't tell her my story just yet. I couldn't move. So I just listened.

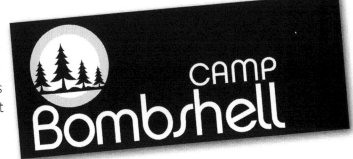

In all my listening, I felt like a fraud. Women come to these camps to share their life experiences and I couldn't bring myself to share mine. I also didn't want to ruin the weekend for some of these women I had grown to love. I wanted things to be as they were, but they couldn't be.

After our talk, I went to my cabin, crawled into my bunk, and pulled the blankets over my head. I couldn't deal with this right now. This was a mistake. I should have stayed home.

Around dinner, I heard Tammi calling my name. I didn't come, but she found me. I remember our conversation word-for-word.

"What are you doing, my friend?"

"I'm hiding," I told her. I was afraid to talk. I was so quiet.

"Hiding from who?"

"Hiding from everyone at camp," I said.

"Why?"

"Coz I felt nauseated. Coz my surgery is two weeks away. Coz I didn't want to tell anyone here and ruin their weekend." The truth was I was scared shitless. I was scared of telling my family I had cancer. I wanted everyone to know and no one to know. How would this all work out?

"And that made you feel like . . ." she said.

"Like hiding and it made me nauseated." Was that really the truth, though?

Tam turned the video camera on her and said, "Because she doesn't want to ruin other people's weekend. Hello. Bombshell, take care of yourself."

"I'm taking care of myself. I'm here."

While Tam was talking, I thought about how I still needed to tell my dad. It was starting to suffocate me that I hadn't told him yet. I was getting even more anxious because I knew that he would not respond in a positive way. If the cancer survival rate chart said that I had a 99 percent chance of making it, he would focus on the one percent chance that I would not. I had to tell him. I was dying a little each day from the silence and thought of how it would break him.

I also worried about the memory it would evoke of Mami. I worried that he would associate her cancer with my own. I worried that he would worry; that he would think I would die just as she did.

I tried to envision the flip side of that coin because I do believe that our thoughts are prayers. And prayers can be manifested. So I thought that this journey of mine would enlighten him. Maybe he would see that I was okay most of the time and that I was coping every day with the support of my friends, family, and doctors.

I thought back to the present again. I thought about the camp and how these women came to escape their own lives, their struggles, and all the stuff they had going on at home. I wanted to be able to provide a nurturing escape for them. I couldn't bring myself to speak my truth: I have cancer, but it would be okay. I looked at Tam and I both hiding in the cabin. How silly we were. Hiding from what? Only our laughter filled the room. That night, I told the campers I was the closest to. It was a huge relief. They nurtured me all weekend and brought me comfort and love. But I still had to tell my dad.

Pat's Journal: May 2, 2008

What wonderful relief. I feel a strange sense of calmness today. Maybe there's nothing wrong with me. I really feel healthy. Maybe a mistake was made and it was someone else's pathology report.

I hung out in the woods by myself a while. I loved being in nature. And that's when I got the call from my doctor telling me that my BRCA Genetic Test results were negative. That means I don't carry the gene. OMG! Thank you. Thank you. Thank you. If I had the gene, I would be at an increased risk of developing ovarian cancer and would have had to have a hysterectomy. I've read that harmful BRCA mutations may also increase a woman's risk of developing cervical, uterine, pancreatic, and colon cancer. It turns out that only an estimated 5 to 10 percent of all female breast cancer cases are hereditary.

I looked everywhere for Tammi and saw that she was on a paddle-boat in the middle of the lake with her daughter Chelsea. I ran to the pier and called out to her. She paddled over to me as I gave her the news, "Got genetic test results! NEGATIVE!"

They paddled over to the dock as quickly as they could. Tammi's daughter jumped out of the paddleboat and hugged me. Tammi looked up and paddled out into the middle of the lake with her arms to the sky thanking God, thanking Spirit. Ten minutes later she paddled over to me and I jumped on the boat and we paddled out together. We cried and hugged and told each other how much we loved one an-other as the sun set into the horizon.

If the results had been positive, I would have needed a hysterec-tomy. An additional surgery was the last thing I wanted, so this was great news. However, had the results been positive, we would have just said, "Oh well. Away with the boobies and the ovaries! Whatever it takes to be healthy."

Pat's Journal: May 8, 2008

I'm finally telling my dad today. It's nine days before my surgery and I've got to tell them soon. I'm so sad to have to do this. My greatest worry throughout this entire process has been gathering the strength to tell my dad. I'm okay. But he's a pessimist. I want him to be able to enjoy his life now. I don't want him to change and become miserable just because of me and what I'm going through. Mercy keeps reminding me that he's my dad and that it's his role to do and be exactly that—take care of me. She's right but at the same time, I have to take into consideration that he's in his seventies and the roles have now been reversed.

Today is the day, but I can't do this alone. I invited Lydia and Annie to join us. We'll all sit down together, drink some wine, and then tell him before we go to dinner.

I drank three glasses of wine before my stepmom and dad arrived. We all sat around the living room drinking. My heart was about to explode through my chest. Lydia and Annie were waiting for my cue. Finally, my dad mentioned an article that came out in the paper that same day referring to genetic testing for breast cancer. Thank you God! Here was my opening.

I said, "Guess what? I had the test a few weeks ago and I'm negative."

He was shocked that I had the test but happy with the results.

I continued quickly without skipping a beat. "But it turns out that I have this really, really tiny little ball that needs to be removed."

My dad and Vivian both froze, as did my heart.

"What? What do you mean a ball?" he said.

"Well . . . a very, very tiny little mass," I said.

Annie chimed in, "Really small, like a grain of rice."

My dad turned to me. "Cancer?"

And with a totally straight and emotionless face, I smiled and said, "Yeah, but it's so tiny that it's no big deal." It was like I was telling him that it was going to rain over the weekend. They were both so stunned that they became numb.

My girlfriends kept the conversation flowing talking about dinner and which restaurant we would go to. Vivian talked about a scare that she had a while back, but my dad just talked about silly stuff. This had gone better than I could have ever imagined, but it was weird. They were too calm and normal—no reaction. We went to dinner, came home, and said goodnight.

The next morning Vivian called to tell me that they had not slept all night. My dad got on the phone and said, "*Las noticias de anoche estaban del carajo.*" (This basically means, "You dropped one hell of a bomb on us last night.")

My heart sank. They were in shock and it hit them when they got home. Vivian told me that my dad cried all night. This is not what I wanted. This was horrible. I need my dad to be okay. Please, dear Lord, bring my father peace. Please bring them both peace.

But the deed was now done. My heart was torn into a million pieces, but now the focus had to be on my healing.

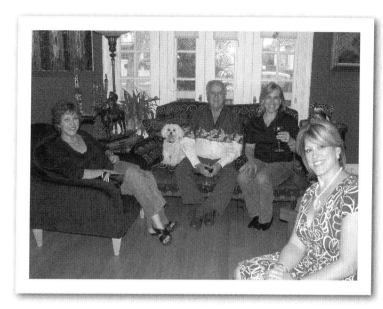

Right before telling my dad and Vivian

Pat's Journal: May 13, 2008

Tammi and I went clothes shopping today. I needed clothes that were loose fitting and buttoned down the front. I had nothing like that in my closet. I went to the maternity department at Target to pick up a few things. It's pretty funny that someone who never had children had to actually look at maternity clothes. One thing's for sure, it's not that simple or easy to find clothes that button down the front or even comes remotely close to being comfortable. I searched for it all . . . PJs . . . shirts . . . dresses . . . you name it. Maybe I should start a clothing line and call it LOOSE.

Pat's Journal: May 16, 2008

The day before my surgery, I took pictures of my breasts. Women should take video or pictures of their breasts before their surgery. After the surgery it will be too late and you can't rewind that tape. It's about no regrets.

I had a long list of things I needed to pack: things to take both to the hospital and to my dad's house. I was actually really calm. My dad and Vivian called to tell me to pack for two weeks. They were so cute: they wanted me to stay with them forever. But I think I'll be okay a few days after the surgery. I was feeling very calm, positive, blessed, and grateful. I hoped I could encourage others to feel the same way.

I heard about a woman who went nuts when she learned she would lose her hair because of chemo. Of course, I didn't want to lose my hair. My hair was very important to me. I want to tell people to be grateful that there are things that can be done to heal us. Look at the positive and focus on that.

I was 24 hours away from my double mastectomy. I was calm and positive. I wanted to get it over with and start treatment. It would be an exciting adventure in life and I knew it would be filled with stories.

I was at my dad's and Vivian's the night before the surgery with Lydia. There was so much love. Lydia was videotaping us, documenting everything: group hugs and lots of love.

So this was what you did on a night before surgery: lots of happiness and celebration. My dad cooked (he ordered Chinese food). It was a joyous night of love. I was so happy. How was this possible?

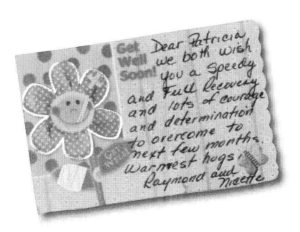

Chapter 10: Time To Rock and Roll

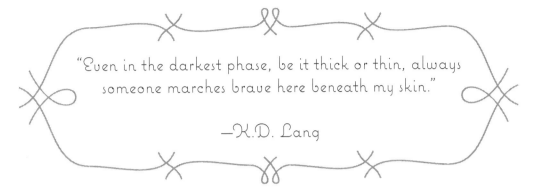

"Even in the darkest phase, be it thick or thin, always someone marches brave here beneath my skin."

—K.D. Lang

The day finally arrived. May 17, 2008. The video camera came into pre-op, too. About 20 of my angels were at the hospital at 6:00 am to wait for my arrival. I arrived with my dad, Vivian, Alex, and Carlos. I brought *Dish & Tell* books for the nurses who wanted all of our signatures.

Pre-op was a riot. Paper panties, a bear paw paper gown and happy juice. My beautiful friends and family lied to me, telling me I looked beautiful in the shower cap and gown.

"I love you guys! Call in all the angels!" I yelled.

I asked the operating room nurse to play my *Sky Spirit* CD, so I could subconsciously hear it. I asked her to please call on all the angels during the surgery, so they could guide the doctors and be with me. She said she would. At that point, I felt my throat tighten and tears begin to well up, but it quickly passed

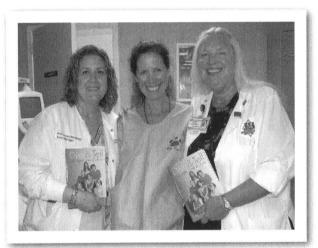

Bombshell fans get their book in pre-op

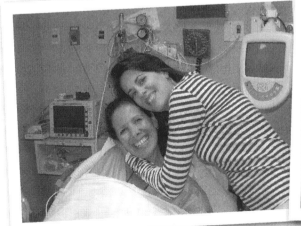

Sweet hugs from Mercy

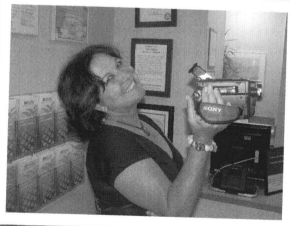

Tammi documenting my journey

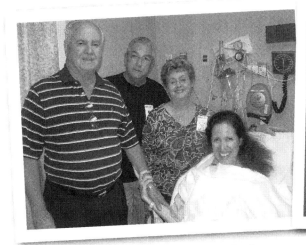
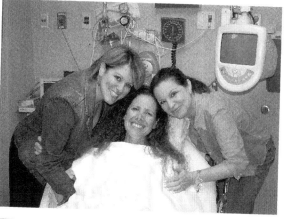

The family prepares for my mastectomy   *Lydia and Maria. Best friends since grade school*

as I reminded myself that this was a beautiful, sacred journey. I was at peace. I had prayed in the morning, wrapping the entire operating room, nurses, doctors, and me in divine white light. This would be a beautiful surgery with wonderful results.

My biggest fear, as usual, was having them find my veins. But the specialist was called in: Mona, my nurse angel. On the first try she found it. *Now*, all was well.

The doctors began arriving. First came Dr. D, with a big, reassuring smile—he was a gem.

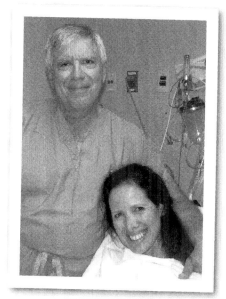

Next the anesthesiologist came followed by the reconstruction surgeon and the doctor who would insert the port. The port was for the administration of the chemo I would receive for a year. He asked me if I wanted the port on my chest or arm.

"Are both the same?" I asked.

Since I was told there wasn't a difference, I opted for the

My hero, Dr. D

arm, figuring it would not show as much. This was a big mistake. I wish someone had explained the differences between the two areas before the day of my surgery.

The happy juice was taking its time working its magic and I was worried because I wanted to be knocked out. As the juice started to take effect, I talked about the Bombshell Musical that was going to premiere the following year.

We videotaped and loved on one another until they wheeled me away.

The surgery took about three hours. I later heard from the nurses that my waiting room was-filled with friends and family. Dr. D came in with the good news. "The cancer was contained," he said. "No lymph nodes involved."

My father finally started to believe that all would be well. Tammi shot him on videotape in the waiting room saying, "I'm very, very, very happy. I was afraid, but the results are good. Now she's gonna be like Dolly Parton."

That's my dad for you. Vivian cried saying, "These are happy tears."

The cancer was contained. My aunt and uncle were overwhelmed with joy.

Kathi formed a prayer circle with everyone there to say thank you. Maria couldn't stop smiling and Lydia and Tammi were in a state of gratefulness.

After the surgery, I cried. My friends cried. I think even the cancer cried. The world rained with tears. My cancer was contained. This was something magical to wake up to. Dr. Marshall had begun the reconstruction procedure right after Dr. D chopped them off.

She put in the expanders that I would need blown up within the next few months. It was now time to reconstruct my body, my breasts, and my newness. It was time to leave the past behind and move forward into a new light, into a new start, and into some new boobies.

Lydia, my ever-present angel, spent the first night with me at the hospital. It's always good to have someone stay over with you.

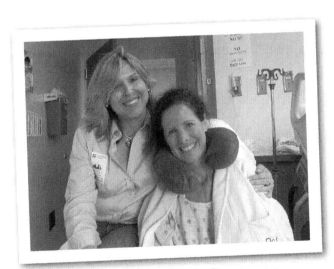

Annie visits me the day after surgery.

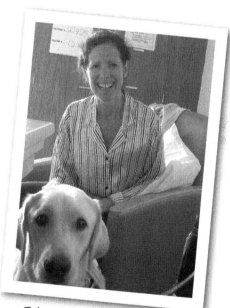

I loved the therapy dog visit

Tammi's Journal: May 18, 2008

It's easy to say it's a journey, a healing process, and sacred. But to actually go thru it, live it, and see it with our own eyes is amazing. It's been quite a learning process for all of us. Pat may have had the actual physical operation, but we've all been operated on these past few days. Pat is walking the talk and she's starting a whole new trend. If you do what she says you should do, it works! Everybody around her is so happy and so calm. We're all so glad to be part of this journey.

Tere, whose family and mine were friends in Cuba before either one of us were born, added:

She's very optimistic. She's always been the person I went to when I felt down in the dumps. I asked myself, "How would Pat feel in this situation?" She is absolutely amazing as far as her optimistic view of life. I'm totally the opposite. I tend to be very pessimistic. She's my role model when I need to feel up.

My biggest problem after the surgery was the shooting pain that would go from the back of my neck and down my left shoulder, elbow, arm, and fingers. It was as if someone was stabbing me in those areas. A physical therapist thought the pain was caused by being in a strange position on the operating table for too long. How bizarre that this was the only pain I was really feeling.

Lydia's Journal, May 18, 2008:

I took a break and sat outside of Pat's room as other visitors came in. After an hour, Pat walked out of the room as if nothing had happened. I was taken aback and laughed. "Who do you think you are? I think you're a fairy. And wow, you look so good!"

I've always had this thing for fairies and all my friends knew that. I even received a life-size Tinker Bell balloon from Tammi that covered my entire hospital window. I loved it!

The most uncomfortable part of the surgery was the drains. They needed to be pinned to your gown and emptied every day depending on how full they got. The fluid needed to be measured to see how much junk was oozing out. It's okay. They didn't really hurt; they were just disgusting. The nurses taught my friends and me how to clean the drains and told us that we needed to squeeze them to make sure there was suction after closing them back up. Gross.

My arm, hand, and neck continued to hurt. It was so weird.

I stayed at my dad and Vivian's for almost a week. They pampered and loved on me. I felt like a little girl back home. It actually felt good. Who wouldn't love being taken care of by such loving people? All I had to do was receive. What a wonderful opportunity I had to spend so much time with them. Why does it take something like this to appreciate what's always been in front of us?

We had visitors every day, although at times I just wanted to rest. Cleaning the drains was a pain. Not literally, just yucky. Lydia learned how to do it. So did a few others but it was always better to have a nurse clean them out. My doctor had ordered a visiting nurse to come to the house every day to clean the drains.

If insurance will pay for that, get it. It puts less stress on you and your caretakers to ensure the drains are cleaned properly.

I couldn't drive, so my friends and family took turns "Driving Miss Daisy's Daughter." Vivian took me to the beauty salon a few days after surgery. Since you can't lift your arms after a mastectomy, I had my long hair shampooed and straightened. Vicky and Annie took me out one afternoon to eat Columbian food and have our usual Cuban *cortaditos*. It felt great to be out and about.

Ten days after my surgery, the drains had to come out. Lydia took me to Dr. Marshall's office. We didn't really know what to expect, so Lydia started to videotape the process as Tina, the nurse, pulled what felt like 500,000 feet of drains from my chest. OMG! I thought the inside of my breast area was being sucked out through the drains. What a horrible, painful ordeal.

How come I wasn't warned? I should have been told to take a truckload of painkillers before coming and that it would hurt like hell. Since then, I've talked with other patients who didn't have this pain. Maybe I had scar tissue build-up and the pulling just tore it up. It didn't matter; I should have taken drugs.

Tammi, Lydia, and I went wig shopping right after the tube removal because Tammi said, "You need to be distracted after the horrible drain-pulling morning."

We were surprised to find that synthetic wigs were the way to go. They were relatively inexpensive and the synthetic hairs were easier to care for. The really cute black wig was $50. Then Lydia bought me a wig that looked just like her hair. We would be twins.

If the doctor gives you a prescription for a cranial prosthesis, the insurance company may cover the cost of the wig.

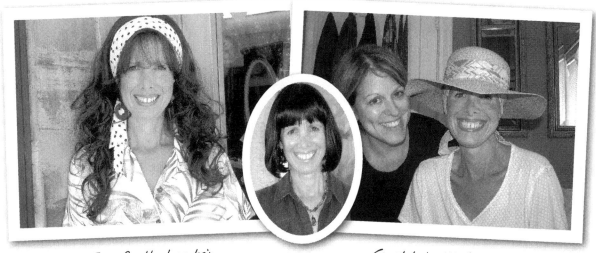

I prefer the long hair   *The Cleopatra look*   *Great hat with bandana*

Tammi's Journal: June 3, 2008

Wow—such an incomprehensible three weeks with Pat after an overwhelming year with my sisters. What is up with all these middle-aged women and breast cancer? All three of my loved ones tested negative on the BRCA Genetic Test, but that doesn't necessarily mean it wasn't inherited. Could it be environmental? Is it the food we're eating? The air we are breathing? It seems everyone I know knows someone who is going through this right now.

Pat sailed through her double mastectomy three weeks ago like the fairy that she is, but this thing with her arm is making me nervous. Something is wrong. The doctors insist it is probably just irritated, so she is having massages and taking painkillers. Her fingers are numb, and she said it feels like bolts of lightning are stabbing her elbow and wrist on a regular basis. The doctors don't want to take it out and move it to her chest, where most ports go. I don't get it.

She's supposed to start chemo in five days but there is no way they are getting anything into that arm. I'm no doctor, but I think she should postpone the chemo till she's got her moving parts in full working order. And if she's not better when we see the on-cologist tomorrow, I'm putting my foot down. I hope he's ready to play Twenty Questions, because I've got them. Pat has no interest in dealing with the details but for better or for worse, I'm becoming a pro at this breast cancer thing. Maybe that's why she put me in charge. It's not like Pat didn't educate herself before she decided to have the radical mastectomy. She spent weeks researching and talking to dozens of women who had walked this path before her. But once the big decisions were made, and the surgery was behind her, she handed the medical baton to us. And we were happy to take it. Pat knows her limits. She needs to put all her energy into enjoying the 'now', staying positive and happy, and enjoying the party-type at-mosphere we're all desperately trying to maintain so she doesn't over-think this.

I'm trying really hard to buy into her positivity, but it's not easy for me to understand how Pat isn't flipping out about the problem with her arm or about the chemo. Even today, when I asked her how she can remain so calm and seemingly happy, and gave her permission to cry (and promised not to tell a soul), she said she had nothing to cry about. I don't get it. How can she be fine? The poor girl's breasts were amputated and now she goes in every few weeks to have her flattened, scarred skin slowly inflated by a plastic surgeon to eventually make room for real implants. Her long, flowing, curly locks are getting cut off next week and we're supposed to celebrate that on camera? We're celebrating everything these days. It seems strange to say this, but we are having a blast just being together, congregating as often as we can in Pat's living room. Sometimes she's napping upstairs and doesn't even know who's there. We're cleaning and scrubbing veggies and cooking and doing laundry so Pat doesn't have to.

We all have our jobs, some more than others. And on top of all of mine, I'm the main videographer of Pat's healing journey.

This video thing is becoming a bit of a circus. Not unusual though since Pat's passion for photography drives most of us crazy. As we videotape her journey though, the deeper we get into this whole cancer thing, the more shocked we are to find so little information out there for people in her shoes. Maybe all the breast cancer swirling around me is happening for a reason. We are being forced to blaze our own trails and with each step, we are gaining more valuable information. That's why we're videotaping all of this—to share what we're learning. If only someone had done that for us.

I organized all my pill bottles two days before my chemo. There was Zantac® (to prevent heartburn) that I took the day before chemo, morning and night; DMX (short for dexamethasone, to prevent nausea and vomiting) that I took the day before, the day of and the day after chemo; and Emend® (three pills for nausea the day before, day of and day after). Each Emend pill was $100. I thought that was crazy. I didn't even know if my insurance would pay for it. Vicky came to help me organize the meds since it was overwhelming. I wrote everything down in my Outlook© Calendar to help me keep my medicine schedule straight.

Then there was the lidocaine cream that I had to remember to take to the hospital. I put that on my calendar too. Another name for this is EMLA Cream®. A friend who went through this told me to put the cream on the port area one hour before going to chemo. The cream would numb the skin. Once I put the cream on, I covered it with Saran™ wrap.

Pat's Journal: June 8, 2008

Chemotherapy starts tomorrow. I know that one of the reasons I'm going through this is because there are a lot of women out there who will benefit from seeing me go through this experience. Tomorrow, I will start receiving healing juices. I can either look at the chemo as something horrific and toxic or I can choose to look at it as sacred juice that is healing me. Modern science is helping me get rid of any unhealthy cells that I might have had in my body. I chose to look at this as something positive and uplifting that comes with a lot of lessons that I'm in the process of learning. The gifts (my family and friends) are just an added bonus, and I have definitely received a lot of them.

I had only one more day until I went for my chemo. I needed an infusion of spirituality so I went to service at Unity on the Bay with a group of girlfriends. We had a delicious lunch with mimosas and then we went to get a manicure and pedicure. Once I began chemo, I had to be careful about getting an infection so I couldn't have manicures until I was finished.

I really wasn't nervous. I was actually anxious about being poked, but not about the chemo. I was ready to get the show on the road.

Chapter 11: Let the Sacred Juice Begin

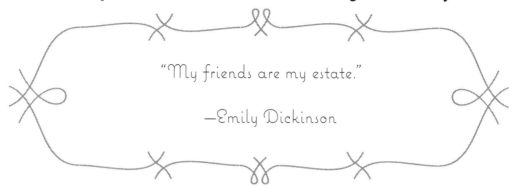

"My friends are my estate."

—Emily Dickinson

On the first day of my chemo, Tere picked me up. We decided to take the longer, scenic route to the hospital and stopped by the Miami River. It was a beautiful morning and I took a moment to breathe.

It's a good idea to be nurtured and pampered before starting treatment. My advice is to disconnect for a few minutes. Be calm so when you go to the hospital, you'll be more relaxed and the chemo will do its work effectively. Tammi was waiting for us when we arrived and Maria arrived a few minutes later. The chemo process is long and you will need to have patience. First, you are checked in. Then they take your blood or review the results of previous blood tests, give you a wristband, ask you questions, and weigh you in. You will then be put in a cubicle to wait for the doctor's order to officially start chemo.

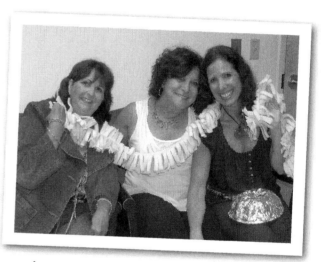

Waiting room with my angels Tammi and Tere

I had fun with my angels and the nurses were awesome. I decided then and there to turn every single chemo treatment into a party. When we finally got comfortable in our cubicle, I created a little sacred space. I took out my mesa that was filled with the stones I had collected from the sacred sites all over the world: the Cavern of the Jaguar in Machu Picchu; Sedona; and the Hawaiian Island of Kauai. In the center I placed the first stone I found at Machu Picchu. I remembered the words of the mystical man who foretold, "You will use this stone to heal yourself and others." I was going to put it to the test.

I also brought a CD player for my Native American flute music. The music was healing for me. Although Tammi thought everything was a bit too out there—or "woo

Chemo 1

← My sacred stone

woo" as she called it—she smiled and played along. I brought a pink boa made for me by Camp Bombshell campers.

It turns out that Orfirio was on vacation that day and I had another nurse. I was bummed about that but once I met my nurse, Awilda, I knew she was wonderful. After being there for almost two hours, the chemo process was about to begin. They first infused me with steroids, Benadryl® and other drugs to help assure that I wouldn't have bad reactions to the chemo and to knock me out. But I was awake, wired, and happy to be there enjoying the company of my friends.

And then, they brought the chemo. The bag was covered in a yellow plastic bag to protect it from the light in the room. I was ready to let the sacred juice begin. I felt nothing. It was just like getting an IV. I was given three types of chemotherapy drugs. First came the Taxotere®.

As it went into my veins, they had me dunk my fingernails and toes in ice water. It seems this specific chemo has a tendency to make your nails brittle and fall off. The ice would prevent the chemo from going there. I asked the nurse, "Can I dump my head in the ice water to prevent my hair from falling out?"

She laughed, "No. It doesn't work."

I felt fine. Maria, Tere, Tammi, and I turned the cubicle into one big party area. Someone came over to us and said, "You ladies have great energy!" We knew that.

When that bag with Taxotere was empty, they ordered the next chemo drug, carboplatin. It took a while before the bag made its way to me, but when it did, the sacred juice continued to flow. After about an hour, the third and final bag arrived: Herceptin®.

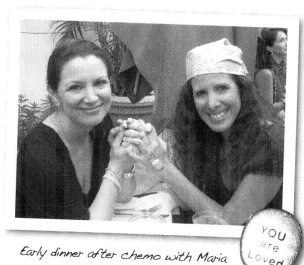

Early dinner after chemo with Maria

YOU are Loved

It was a good day. All those bad cells were getting killed off.

Pat's Journal: Week of June 9, 2008

Day 1: Chemo felt like nothing. The pre-drugs made me a little light-headed, but they didn't put me out as they did to most everyone in the cubicles around me.

Day 2: Today I got a Neulasta® shot in the stomach. It didn't hurt. This shot is to build up my white blood count and to help me avoid infection. I feel fine. It's given 24 hours after every chemo treatment.

Day 3: I am a bit tired and a little queasy today.

Day 4: Today I am a bit queasier and a little more tired.

Day 5: I napped all day. Of all the days, today I was the most tired. Today's stool was soft.

Day 6: Today's stool was really soft but I felt less queasy.

Day 7: Today's stool was soft as well. I felt a little less queasy. I ate more. Last night I had more diarrhea than I care to comment on (maybe chocolate ice cream cake didn't help). I took imodium and it stopped. Strange smells and tastes started. I tasted something metallic on my tongue and I had dry mouth and rectal irritation. TMI, I know.

The next two weeks were okay. I gained strength every day. This chemo wasn't so bad.

Pat's Journal: July 1, 2008

I've discovered mouth sores. What should I use for this? Overall, I'm good during the day. I'm getting diarrhea again at night. I took imodium and hot tea. Okay, so far so good. Still haven't thrown up yet. Feels like I have a cold. Guess those are the cold-like symptoms you sometimes get. My throat is a bit scratchy and sore. I'm beginning to get chills, but not so bad. Port has to go! Too much pain in the arm.

Tammi's Journal: June 29, 2008

It's almost three months since the Big C diagnosis, with one chemo treatment down and 16 more to go. But only five of the really strong treatments left. Pat has become an expert at turning lemons into lemon drops, and while a handful of us are doing our best to keep Pat happy, entertained, and well-fed, I have to go out of town for a few weeks and I'm a little worried about leaving her.

The first ten days after chemo is called NADIR. I looked it up and it refers to the blood counts, particularly white blood cell count and platelet count. NADIR basically means low point, when your immune system is most suppressed. Believe it or not, something as plain as sliced turkey from the deli can make her sick, so we rotate scrubbing veggies and shopping and cooking organically for her.

Chapter 12: Hair Today, Bald Tomorrow

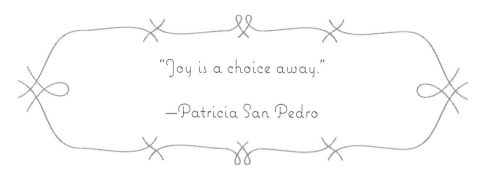

"Joy is a choice away."

—Patricia San Pedro

I knew the day would come when I would have to cut my hair. The doctors suggested cutting it off before it started to fall out in clumps. My hair had always been an important part of me. It was big and long and crazy and it was me.

So, it seemed like a good idea to have a hair-cutting party. I invited my girlfriends to my house and Chip from the *Scott Alan Salon.* I needed a friend to cut off my hair. My friend Liza was appointed as the Locks of Love representative since I wanted to donate my hair. She found their website (**www.LocksofLove.org**) and learned the hair had to be at least ten inches long, washed, dried, tied in a ponytail, and cut right above the hairline.

I thought I was prepared but I suddenly felt overwhelmed. Somehow I was dealing better with losing my breasts than losing my hair. It took a few minutes to get past the emotion and then I wanted to just get it over with. My friends held my hand as Chip did the deed. The first words out of my mouth were "That didn't hurt at all."

I looked at myself in the mirror and laughed. It was all very strange. Chip cut it shoulder-length first, before cutting it all the way. A little at a time was all I could handle. I looked like a poodle, but everyone loved it.

After I cut my hair, I finally gave in and had my port surgically removed since the pain wasn't going away. They took the port out of my arm and placed it on my chest near where the bra

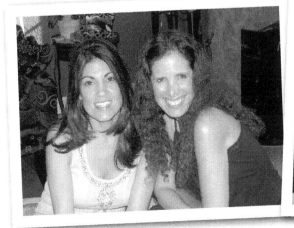

Before the haircut with my friend Jade

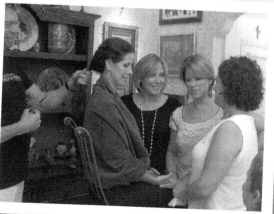

Here it goes . . .

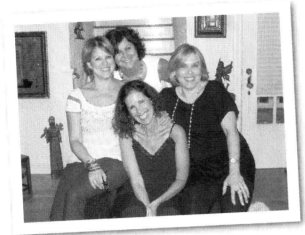

Halfway there

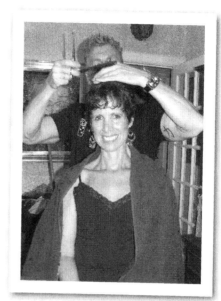

Here comes the poodle look

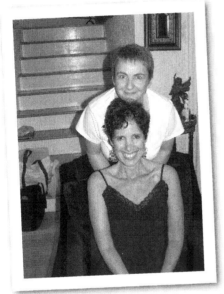

My friend Liza with hair shorter than mine

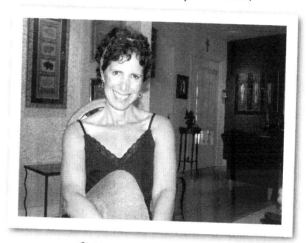

Getting used to short hair

strap goes. After surgery, the doctor said that it would never have gotten better. It was right on top of the median nerve and it was totally irritating it. Tammi was right all along. I should have removed it from my arm a long time ago. But now I was ready for my second chemo session and could receive my sacred juice through my port.

Pat's Journal: June 30, 2008

Judy is flying in today to take me to chemo. I am so excited and feel so loved and blessed. My sweet Judy. We've been friends for more than twenty-five years. We're totally different. She's a country girl and calls me a city mouse. But she's a soul sister.

My brand new port worked! What a breeze. I was so happy it didn't hurt at all when they put the needle in. The lidocaine numbed it. The sacred juice was flowing, doing its beautiful work in my body. Any and all unhealthy cells in my body were being left behind with only good, clean, wholesome healthy cells staying in place. Due to scheduling conflicts, Orfirio was still not my chemo nurse but I would get him yet!

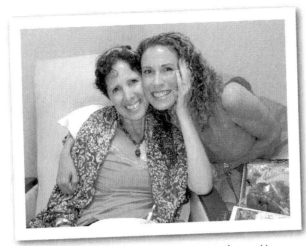

Sweet Judy came from New Hampshire

As I sat through my second chemo session, I observed others receiving chemo. I noticed their relationships with those who accompanied them. Some were with family members and some were alone. Some were young and some were old. I began to have many thoughts. I thought about creating a non-profit that manages Angels—caregivers that can accompany patients to treatments. I also thought that the hospital should assign candy stripers or staff to cruise the treatment area and make patients happy, maybe with an arts and crafts cart like when I had my breast surgery.

At exactly seven minutes after I wrote down these ideas, I began to feel a pressure on my chest and my stomach started hurting. My face turned beet red and I had trouble breathing. These symptoms happened within ten seconds of each other. Judy saw me and ran to get the nurse who immediately turned off the IV. I was having an allergic reaction to the chemo drug Taxotere®. I found out that it is not uncommon for some patients to get an allergic reaction to this drug the second time they receive it. So why wasn't I warned, monitored more closely, or given additional pre-meds?

As soon as the IV stopped, I was okay again. The reaction subsided, but I was still scared. Thank goodness Judy was there with me. I'm not sure I could have called out for help on my own. I realized once again how vital it was for someone to be there with you during each and every chemo treatment.

After the reaction, the nurse called my doctor and they ordered extra Benadryl® and decadron. I was still scared. I waited 30 minutes after each dose before starting the Taxotere again at a slower rate. This time it went well.

I resumed my observation of the other patients. An older, very frail woman in the cubicle next to me didn't look very happy. After a while, a woman in a business suit walked in and sat beside her. She pulled her laptop out and started typing. There was absolutely no interaction.

Across from me, a mom was waiting with her thirty-year-old daughter who was about to get chemo. Perhaps her mother was thinking that it's not supposed to be this way—that it should be her, not her daughter, in that chair. Both mother and daughter were talking and smiling at each other. They were caught in the embrace of love. Mom smiled at her daughter and it was as if she was saying without any words, *It will be okay. I am here.* I looked at the older woman in the cubicle next door with the woman I assumed was her daughter. I wished there was more communication, but who was I to judge?

What I have learned through this experience is that sharing stories and reflecting on experiences is what promotes healing and recovery. I've become a collector of stories from the people closest to me.

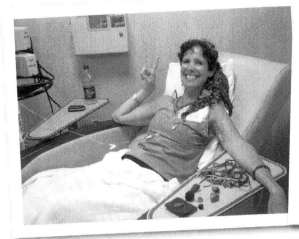
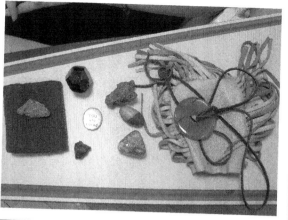

Sacred juice begins   *My sacred stones. Always with me at chemo*

Judy's story:

I flew from New Hampshire to Miami as soon as I could to be with Pat to help her through round two of chemotherapy. Medications throughout the day caused her to jumble her thoughts and words. At one point she pointed to her apple juice saying "Oh, my apple sauce melted!" Realizing her confusion, we exploded with laughter. Throughout the day she blew kisses to patients, signed copies of her book, ***Dish & Tell,*** for the staff, wrote in her journal, meditated, and blessed each strand of hair as it toppled from her head. We speculated about whom she would look like when it grew back. Cleopatra? Madonna? It was just one more thing for Pat to look forward to.

That night, Pat slept well on the new red satin pillowcases Tammi and Lori had given her. The pillowcases would help slow down the hair-shedding process and ease her scalp sensitivity.

Pat subsequently had a fabulous week filled with tremendous energy and presence. We've laughed about her new, now very short, hairdo and inventoried her assortment of wigs and turbans. Short naps offered renewed strength for errands and visits from friends. We were all amazed at Pat's resilience. We took advantage of her energy and appetite, knowing that days following chemotherapy could be slightly difficult. We've enjoyed delicious food (homemade by well-wishers from as far away as Alabama), brief trips downtown to her favorite bookstore and Cuban café, DVD movies at home, and late-night chats. My visit sadly came to an end on Tuesday when Kathi came by to spend the day with Pat after they took me to the airport.

Flying home I reflected on the joyousness of this visit and Pat's incredible resolve. She savored each delicious moment of being, existing, feeling, and finding promise and hope with every passing second. Meanwhile, she's learning to receive the help and gifts of love and friendship that are coming her way.

She is in awe of the many people who have reached out to her and is humbled by the incredible messages sent to her on **CarePages**. Pat has embarked on an incredible, life-altering healing journey. I am changed by her strength and courage. She reminds us that attitude carves our path throughout life and that we have great choices available to us.

Pat's Journal: July 2, 2008

No side effects to this chemo at all. It's a beautiful thing! Hopefully it will last through the 4th of July weekend so I can have some fun.

Tammi's Journal: July 5, 2008

Pat feels like shit today. Again five days after chemo seems to be the worst. She's exhausted and although we did our best to make it a Happy 4th of July, positioning my living room couches right in front of the window to watch fireworks without lifting even our heads off the pillows, my poor friend was exhausted. But she's still happy. Pat knows in the deepest part of her soul that to experience pleasure, you must first experience pain. It's the most primal theory, but I never really knew anyone who actually bought into it.

She is truly living in the right now, and enjoying every moment, especially because she is surrounded by so much love. And so each day becomes a new adventure with fun-filled field trips sandwiched between doctor appointments. There are about 15 rotating angels—all friends who merely ask "What can we do?"—and, unlike most people who retreat and don't resurface till their hair is grown back in, Pat takes each one of us up on our offer. She has learned the important gift of receiving.

Talking about my cancer and sharing it with my friends and family has given me a new perspective of relationships. By providing them with the opportunity to participate in my healing journey, I can encourage a healing space for them and me. Cancer does not have to be a solitary experience.

Chapter 13: Doing the Chemo Conga

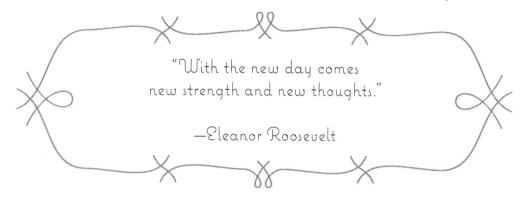

"With the new day comes new strength and new thoughts."

—Eleanor Roosevelt

As chemo three approached, some of my friends were on vacation, others were busy, and some of them even forgot about my food for the week. I know that it's my responsibility, but since I've been taken care of during the previous two chemo treatments, I didn't think about it until it came time to eat and there wasn't much in my fridge. I slept alone for the first time since chemo began and visits from my friends were now sporadic. I missed the attention. I missed being taken care of, especially since I've been exhausted the last two days and I've had to fend for myself. *What a spoiled rotten brat I've become,* I thought. Maybe I took this learning to receive a bit over the top. My wonderful friends probably spoiled me without realizing it and now it was hard to be alone. I woke up alone. I ate breakfast alone. When I worked, I worked from home and spent most of my day alone. I ate lunch in front of the computer. And then, unless my dad and stepmom or a girlfriend called me up to get together, I ate dinner alone. Then I went to bed alone.

Enough, I thought. It was time to grow up. But it was also part of the reality of living by myself. For some reason, this was beginning to sadden me.

I was also bored. I didn't go out much. There wasn't much work to do. I had two potential clients that I was going to meet with next week. Although I was excited about the financial potential, I was scared because I was not sure how much I could focus or how creative I could be. I had my own company with one employee—*me!* I had never wanted my job to consume me. I had lived in the corporate world for too long and I was not going there again. Having a little boutique firm with a few trusted outsourced professionals was all I wanted.

But now, if I was tired or not feeling well, I had a problem because I couldn't be creative if my mind was mush and I was exhausted. I couldn't be out there networking to attract new clients.

My bank account was dwindling and my bills were increasing. There were pills that insurance had not paid for yet and bills rejected by insurance.

I began to think, *Am I going to have to work until the day I die? Will I be able to retire? Will I find a soulmate? Who will take care of me when my friends are too busy?* Wow. The thoughts that popped into my brain when I had nothing better to think about.

Would I find my soulmate? I realized my soul was the most important part of me, but I was feeling like my physical features were more important to attract a potential mate. I was 52 years old, bald, no nipples, breasts were under reconstruction, I had a history of breast cancer, and I was flabby with cellulite. Why would *ANY* man want me versus someone else with prettier packaging? I was officially having my first pity-party.

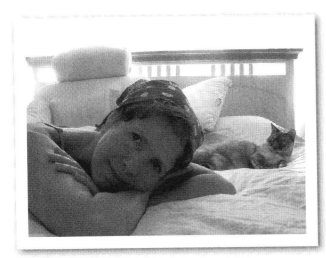

Bored at home

I wished I had a partner in my life to hold me in his arms when I fell asleep, to eat dinner and cuddle with in front of the television, to take me to the movies or dancing when I was feeling up to it, or to just say good morning to when I opened my eyes. I welcomed a partner who didn't have to put the rest of his life on hold in order to see me, because I would be the rest of his life.

Friday night. All my friends were either out or with their families. Good for them. with my cat and my laptop and felt sorry for myself.

I wanted so bad to be creative, to come up with great ideas and concepts to change the world, to help other women going through this, but at that moment my brain was mush and my pity party was in full-swing. It was the weekend before my next chemo, which meant my immune system was at its best. I wanted to go out and have fun. But there was no one to do it with.

I started the expansion process. It wasn't a big deal at all. Lydia and I went to Dr. Marshall's office. I had spread lidocaine cream over the two expander port areas so I wouldn't feel the needle going in. Tina took about 20 seconds per breast. She stuck a little needle into the expander port which I didn't feel and then pumped saline into it. It was quick and painless as I saw my breasts begin to grow. It was actually very cool.

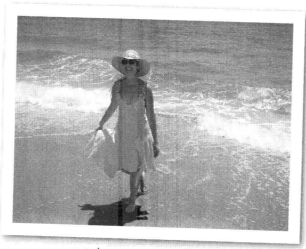

Quick escape before chemo

I told Tina early on that I didn't want to rush the process. I was in no hurry and I didn't want it to hurt. I would probably need to go in every month for about six months to get me to a full C-cup size.

My first expansion was done. It was a breeze and I could already see cleavage. Yay!

Mark flew into town to take me to my third chemo session. Lydia would meet us there and finally, Orfirio would be my chemo nurse!

The sacred juice started to pump into my veins at about nine o'clock that morning. Lydia was nowhere to be found. She's usually late for everything, but I didn't think she'd be late for chemo. We called her. She said that the cupcakes she was baking burned and she was baking new ones. *WHAT?* I told her I didn't care about the cupcakes but really just wanted her here. She said she would hurry.

At 1:00 pm, Lydia arrived with trays of cupcakes. I knew her too well. She didn't want to be here. This was too difficult for her and the baking was just an excuse. I told her I was fine and all was well.

With tears in her eyes she said, "Instead of you calling it chemo, you call it sacred juice. You have your stones, you believe, you meditate. But it's all attitude. It's all in the mind. You're receiving chemo and going through this whole thing with such a great attitude. And you're sitting here, comforting me!"

It turned into a funny moment.

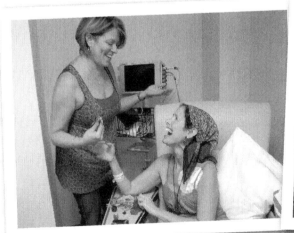
Sharing a laugh with Lydia

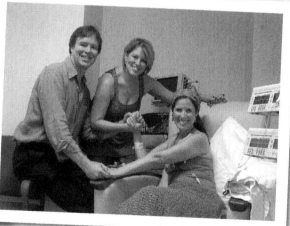
Chemo 3 with Mark and Lydia

I explained to her that a part of my recovery was confronting fear and accepting the fear as something unknown; accepting that I might not know everything that will happen and being totally okay with that. I had to give up control. That was a challenge since I always thought I was in control. I decided to not fight my fear, but to embrace it and accept it as something I could learn from.

Pat's Journal: July 25, 2008

Four days after chemo, Mark flew back to Dallas. I slept fourteen hours last night. I just couldn't bring myself to do anything other than wrap myself in my comforter and sheets with Pucci at my feet and call it a night; a long night. It felt good! I've learned to do what my body asks and I am blessed to be able to do that. If it's hungry, I feed it. If it's not, I don't.

I'm really doing amazingly well on this chemo cruise. Every three weeks I hop on that ship. I take time off from work (well, there isn't much work) and relax. Sure it's not the kind of vacation I would actually plan, but if I look at it this way, it makes it a bit more appealing and less daunting.

I was doing great other than becoming forgetful. Chemo brain was setting in. It's a very real side-effect from the treatment. I would completely forget words or say one word when I meant another. Not the usual forgetfulness that comes with menopause—it's different. I would say things like "fart" instead of "party."

One angel leaves and another arrives. Gilda was a camper who came to one of our Camp Bombshells. Since then, we have traveled to a spiritual retreat in Peru and have become very close friends.

Gilda's Story:

I could not wait to jump on the highway and head down from Palm Beach to Coral Gables to spend some time with Pat! This weekend was finally my turn to spend time with her.

When I arrived I was expecting to find an optimistic Pat but also a tired, maybe sleepy or "I am not hungry" version of Pat. But what did I see when I pulled up to her house? A beautiful Pat, very short hair with a scarf worn as a headband in a long summer dress, walking her dog Merlot down the street! Her skin looked fresh: no makeup, no bags under her eyes, and no wrinkles. She looked rested and glowing!

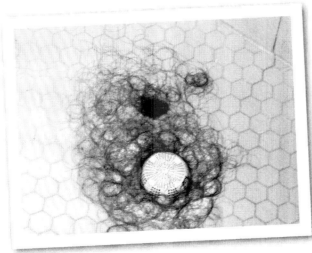

Drain with my hair

Saturday she woke up and washed her hair. She had been putting it off for four days, knowing that a lot of what she had left would literally go down the drain. And it did. She even took a picture. But remarkably, she still has hair after several chemo treatments. It's unusual, but her doctor said that it certainly will all fall out shortly. She said it was way too thin for her to go out in public so Saturday became her first wig day.

We shared an evening with wine (her doctor said one or two was okay) and a good old movie—brand-new for the two of us: Urban Cowboy. We loved it as well as the very hot John Travolta! Perfect chick flick for the girls!

Annie and Vicky joined us for breakfast the next morning and we planned our post-chemo girls' trip to Santorini, France, and Italy. When I said good-bye, I did it with a happy heart, having shared a wonderful time with my friend and seeing how well she was doing. I personally witnessed how having a positive attitude can turn a very difficult experience into a positive life-changing one.

Pat's Journal: August 10, 2008

Tomorrow is chemo number four which means I'm more than half-way there with the big chemo drugs. That powerful sacred juice! I'm feeling physically great, thankfully. Yesterday I woke up at 6:30 a.m. and spent hours running errands with Annie. I was filled with energy without even taking a nap. When we were done, I came home and did more stuff around the house . . . hanging up paintings, moving furniture around, putting up decorations on my new shelves, etc. By midnight, I was pooped so I went to bed.

Annie and Tammi took me to chemo 4. Orfirio was my nurse so we had a blast.

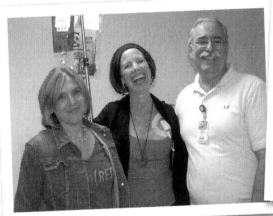
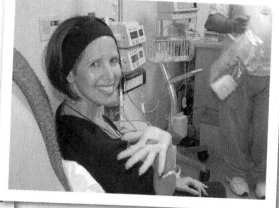

Having a blast with my nurse and Annie

My sacred stone from Peru

It was Annie's first time being with me at chemo. She was very emotional.

I was nauseous and felt sick. I had to cry a little bit. It was scary. I still can't believe that Pat has cancer. And I know that it's because she doesn't eat Oreos®! Seriously, though, I love Pat so I had to be here. I didn't know what it was going to be like. She looked great and wasn't vomiting. She was at peace. What does she call it? Sacred juice? It's good.

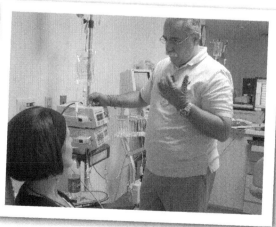

Orfirio answers all my questions

Chemo went well. We were there for about five hours so it was a relatively short day.

By day three, four, or five after my chemo session, I would start to get tired. I was never sick to my stomach or ill the way my mom was ill. The current medications are amazing, so there was no need at all for fear.

However, with chemo number four, it was hard to get out of bed. Just making breakfast was a challenge and at times it took me up to two hours to get up enough strength to do this. This was one of the challenges of living alone. But I saw each of these moments as a chance to learn about this experience.

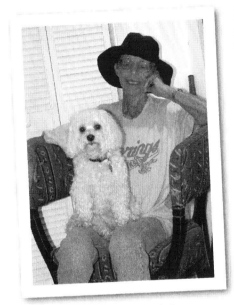

Kathy and Merlot

I made myself some waffles and a smoothie with fresh strawberries and blueberries that my friends had cleaned. The fruit needed to be clean because my immune system was very sensitive during chemo. If you have family and friends and you live alone, just have them help you clean your produce so you can prepare your food on your own. My wonderful neighbor and friend Kathy across the street walked Merlot every day that week. I didn't really have the strength to do it.

The rest of the three weeks that followed were uneventful. I was tired, but little by little I got my strength back. Friends and family visited from time to time and I spent my time doing pretty much nothing. I didn't even journal. I gave myself permission to vegetate. It was boring at times since I lived alone, but I made the best of it. My babies Merlot, Tango, Chloe, and Pucci always kept me company.

Tammi's Journal: August 30, 2008

As time goes on and Pat soars through her treatments, the angels were flying back into their own lives. Human nature, I guess. My sister said the worst part of her cancer was when she started to feel better and all her chicks flew the coop.

Last night, Pat commented that if she had a husband, siblings, or even a boyfriend, everyone would have just assumed she

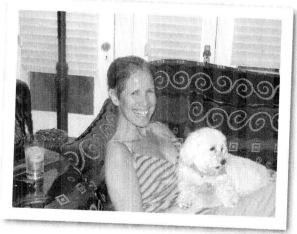

Merlot loves me with or without hair

was well taken care of and left her to recuperate with relatives. She might not have had the chance to be surrounded by so much love.

I worry about Pat because I'm afraid she has taken this "I'm fine, I'm grateful for my cancer" bit a little too far. I'm just afraid that when she does feel horrible, she won't share that with a soul because she is so focused on remaining positive. She believes that giving into the sadness or pain or nausea will make her psychologically weak. If you ask me, no matter how spiritual a being you are, being nauseous and dizzy and in pain day after day has got to get to you. I only hope that pushing all those feelings down and mustering up a smile is not doing any damage to her body inside.

But every day she tells me she's not sick any more, just tired. And that the cancer is out of her and a little discomfort is the price you pay for "insurance" as she calls it. I hope she's being true to herself because she's got nothing to prove to me.

What a gift to be able to constantly see the blessings of adversity. Most people who have cancer see this when the fight is over, but to be weathering the storm without a compass and never even flinching when entering uncharted, possibly deadly waters is incredible to witness. Either she has figured out a way to completely disconnect herself from her new reality or she's a robot. I haven't decided. She really should have cracked by now, and although she's exhausted and a little shocked at how this insidious disease (and its treatments) has taken over her life, she's really living in the moments of joy that come when she's feeling loved, and that's what keeps her spirits up.

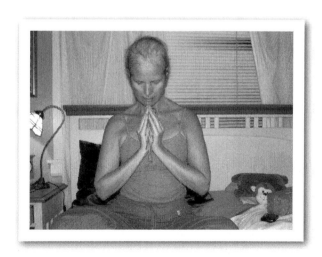

Meditating at home

Chapter 14: Last of the BIG Ones

"When the Japanese mend broken objects, they aggrandize the damage by filling the cracks with gold. They believe that when something's suffered damage and has a history it becomes more beautiful."
—Barbara Bloom

I wore one of my fun wigs on September 1 as I headed to my fifth chemo session with Stefanie and Maria. My white blood count was a little low, but I was eating lots of yummy lentils with beef that Lydia and Mercy had cooked for me. I was going to feel good after this. Once today was over, I would have one more major chemo session and then I would take Herceptin®. I heard that the side effects from Herceptin were easier to deal with than the chemo side effects.

As I was getting this sacred juice, I felt a calm come over me. I felt no different than if I wasn't having chemo put inside my veins. As usual, the actual infusion of chemotherapy was no big deal.

I always brought my healing sacred stones with me to every session and I always prayed before coming to chemo as a way to open up my sacred space. I prayed that all of this would be wonderful and healing and nurturing. I told everything that shouldn't be in my body to leave and go the other way. I said, "Thanks for the visit and the lessons; now go on your merry way." I was protecting my healthy cells so they wouldn't get nuked.

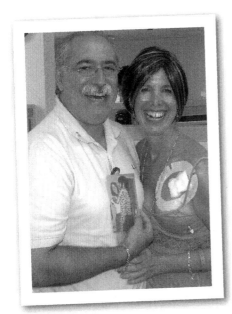

Orfirio and me . . . then and now

Stefanie said:

Fear, whether it is fear of chemo, death, or anything in your life, is taking away so much from your daily experiences. I think that fear is the worst part of whatever you're going through. The "going through" is never as bad as the fear you have. They also say the diagnosis is always worse than the disease. From my experience, nothing is as bad as I feared. The experience is better. Don't be afraid.

I brought pictures of Orfirio and me from 26 years ago. We shared them with all the nurses and they couldn't believe it was him.

The date was September 22, 2008. It was five o'clock in the morning and I was getting my last big time chemo session in three hours. My friend Anne (from camp) had flown in from New Jersey yesterday to be with me for the big day tomorrow. But I couldn't sleep. I watched episodes of *Sex in the City, Will and Grace,* and *American Idol.* I burned sage, prayed and played loud music. I couldn't shut off my brain. I was so tired, but I was ready to get this done so I could move on.

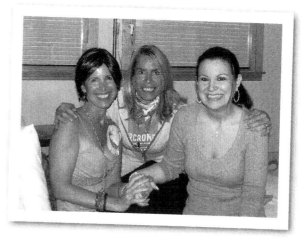

My angels Stefanie and Maria

I had been calling cancer a gift, but was it really a gift? Gifts are given to you by people who want to make you happy. Perhaps it was an opportunity to review and reflect on my life. Did I get the lessons I should be learning? How was I going to do everything I had to do after cancer? What was the reason behind this all? I looked up at the clock: 5:20 am. I had to get up at seven to go to chemo. I was already up.

Mercy called me. "So, how are you feeling?"

"I feel fabulous. I only slept for forty minutes last night. I was anxious about all this stuff," I said.

"You worried about insurance?" asked Mercy.

"I'm worried about insurance. I'm worried about money. I have one client left who goes away in two weeks. I watched TV, burned sage, prayed, and ate Weight Watchers®' popsicles."

"I want to know why you're eating Weight Watchers at this point in your life!"

"Because I eat a lot of them and because I've gained thirteen pounds and they taste delicious."

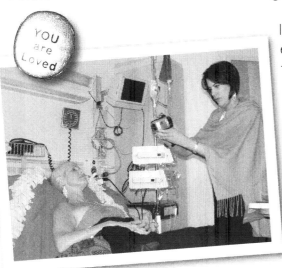

I showered and dressed and wore my chandelier earrings. You can't really be vain going through this process but I couldn't help myself. I had to maintain some type of glamour.

I left with Anne to go to chemo. Mercy and Tammi joined us there. Mercy and I brought our mesas with us. I was tired when I arrived at chemo. I had not slept all night and this time the pre-meds made me sleepy. Mercy picked up the video camera and captured a moment on tape.

Mercy takes over videotaping duties

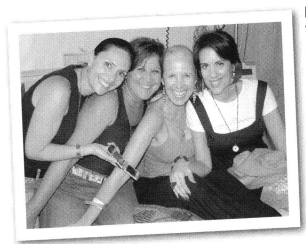

Chemo party with my angels

I woke up about an hour later feeling refreshed. We had such a fun day. We laughed and told stories of all the crazy things we did at Camp Bombshell.

I was on my third chemo bag and it was getting closer to the end. *Thank you, Spirit. Thank you, Angels. Thank you, God!*

Anne was getting the video camera ready. Drum roll . . . and that was it. I was done. Anne took a picture of the empty chemo bag. I was so grateful. It was the last of the milky fluid, the liquid gold. The sacred juice had finished going through my veins. That was it. That was it.

Mercy and Tammi hugged me. "It is the end," they said. "Anne, look at that empty bag. Oh my God!"

The IV bell rang and rang indicating it was all over. I picked up the phone and called my dad and other angels. "Do you hear that noise? Do you know what it is? That's the end of chemo! Yay! Is that not the most beautiful sound?" I had to share that magical moment. Now it was time to celebrate."

I still had six more months (11 sessions) of Herceptin left. But that would be easier. My white blood count would start to go up. During chemo, I wasn't supposed to be around too many people because of possible infection. I also had to be careful of being in public places such

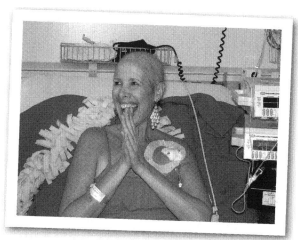

I'm so happy

as theaters, restaurants, and planes. I did everything possible to stay healthy and I was lucky enough to not get a cold or anything. But now that the major chemos were done, I needed a break. I had been home for five months. I was ready to get away for a bit. I could travel wherever I wanted to go.

I decided to throw my angels a party. I could never repay what they've done and continue to do for me, but I had to try. So, a party was a good start.

We gathered at a fun restaurant in Miami. I got angel wings for my archangels, Lydia and Tammi, and we celebrated the night away.

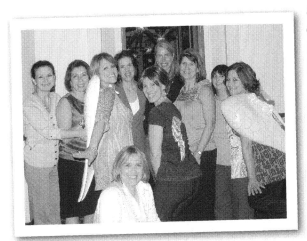

Angel gathering

Two weeks later, I celebrated by going to my log cabin in North Carolina with Lydia, Maria, and her sister Dianita. Before take-off, I remembered to grab my lymphedema sleeve. A lymphedema sleeve is like a tight girdle for the arm. It stretches all the way up to the shoulder and covers the entire arm. This is supposed to prevent the buildup of lymphatic fluid. I didn't have any infected lymph nodes and only one node was surgically removed, but I decided to wear one for preventative measures. I had heard that about 33 percent of women who have had breast cancer surgery get lymphedema and I wanted to do everything possible to avoid this.

Lydia called me the "masked lady" since I wore a surgical mask. But I wasn't about to take any chances. I just had chemo about two weeks before and there were a lot of germs on a plane. So I ate my bagel and then put my mask on. I was ready to take off.

As I sat on the plane with my friends, I felt such gratitude to be alive and to be healthy. Being diagnosed with cancer was a hard path and a constant struggle. But I wasn't alone. It was important to see the goodness even when it was difficult, even when I felt that I would fall apart into tiny pieces and scatter.

I spent a magical week in North Carolina celebrating life. It was the closest we had ever been. Never before had we appreciated each other as much as we did now. Cancer was a reminder that every day was a gift.

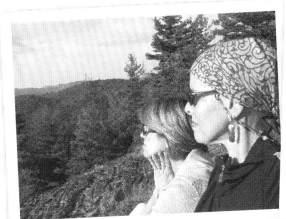
Enjoying nature with Lydia

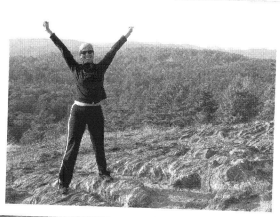
Celebrating life

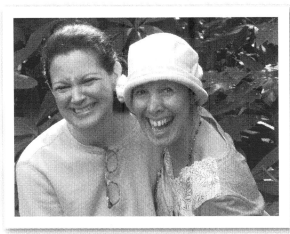
Loving life with Maria

When I returned, I spent time making television and radio station appearances. It was Breast Cancer Awareness Month and I wanted to get the word out: early detection, talk to your doctor, and if you have dense breasts, you need more than a mammogram.

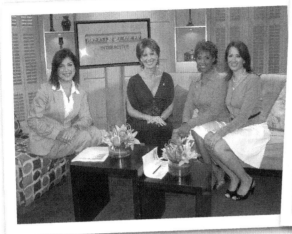

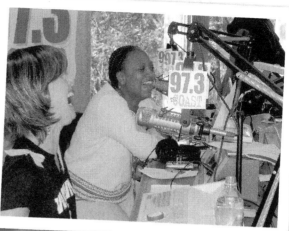

Breast Cancer Awareness Month on NBC 6

97 The Coast with the Two Girls in the Morning Show

Finally, I decided to shave my head. I had convinced myself that I looked okay with my thin wisps of hair. The reality was that I looked sick. Once it was shaved, I actually looked pretty cool.

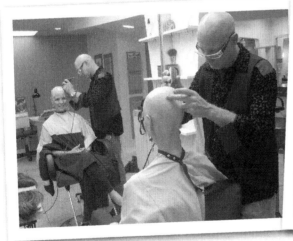

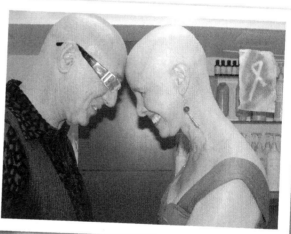

Scott Alan takes it all off

Two bald peas in a pod

Chapter 15: New Breasts For the Holidays

"You can't change the past,
but you can ruin a perfectly good present
by worrying about the future."
—Anonymous

This holiday season was going to be the best ever. Gratitude was ever-present, every moment of the day. Never had Thanksgiving meant so much.

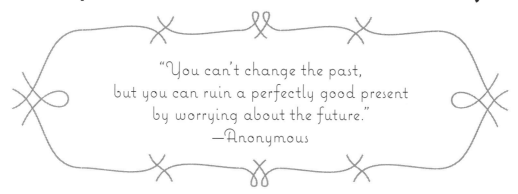

Sweet cousins

My cousins and godsons

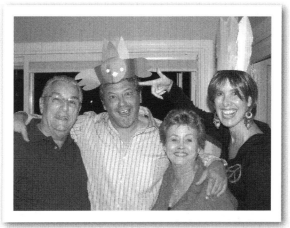

Silly fun with my family

Santa was about to bring me brand new C-cup breasts. I was so excited. After all of my fill-ups, I was now ready to get my boobies. The expanders would come out and the permanent implants would go in. My implants were going to be filled with half silicone and half saline.

Off I went, back to South Miami Hospital where the nurses I knew all too well greeted me with open arms. My dad, Vivian, and Lydia accompanied me.

Dr. Marshall marked me up right before surgery and we talked about my size C cup and the color of my tattooing for the areola. She would start the process during surgery but finish it off later at her office. It was like picking paints for your house. I looked through a color palette and picked out the color of my areola. What a strange new reality this was.

I went home after the surgery feeling a bit woozy from the anesthesia. It was back to recovering: no lifting, no driving, and just chilling.

About a week or so later, it was time for the great unveiling. Lydia picked me up and we went to Dr. Marshall's office where Tina would remove the bandages.

We were all excited to see my new breasts. Already I could tell they looked great. Dr. Marshall was an artist and I was loving the cleavage I saw under the wrapping. I decided not to look down as Tina started the process. Lydia was videotaping. She first removed the bandage from the side that did not have the cancer. I looked at Lydia's face as she looked at my new breast and nipple. I didn't like what I saw. Her expression told me she was trying to smile while inside she was about to throw up.

Tina assured us that the alien on my breast called a nipple would soon look normal. It was in-flamed and raw.

And then I was taken over the top. As the second breast was uncovered, I looked down to see *no nipple! What?* OMG! I was deformed. It was the first time during this entire process that I felt deformed.

Tina assured us that everything would be fine in the end. Sometimes the skin is too tight on the breast that had cancer and it takes several tries to build a nipple. This would be a simple procedure in the doctor's office. Tina explained that Dr. Marshall was a perfectionist and didn't want to risk tearing the skin.

I'm good with that. I understand. But I didn't know. I thought I would be coming here and welcoming two brand new perfectly assembled breasts with nipples. It was the not knowing and the surprise that literally made me almost vomit.

We left in a hurry. We were both ill to our stomachs. I had an alien on one breast and no nipple on the other.

Would I ever be normal again?

Pat's Journal: December 14, 2008

The week from hell. I looked at my new breasts to see that I only have one nipple and the other one is a being from another planet. Yes, of course, eventually there would be two, but it is hard for me to describe the feeling right now that I have in the pit of my stomach.

Pat's Journal: December 18, 2008

Bare Truths

Today I posed topless for the second time in front of two men I barely knew. It was my second nude photo shoot in less than a month. No, I wasn't getting paid, and you won't see the pictures in any centerfold. Heaven forbid.

It was embarrassing, humiliating, and emotionally painful. I felt deformed and with no sense of femininity or sensuality. For better or for worse, I am sporting a newly built, grotesquely swollen raw nipple on one breast, no nipple on the other, and two very ugly scars from my mastectomy. Most people would do everything possible to hide these puppies.

But taking these pictures is the only way for me to authentically show others what my journey has been like in full, raw, living color.

So there I stood, bare-chested in a television production studio's garage, surrounded by very bright lights aimed at my breasts, and two men who barely knew me, doing me the favor of shooting me, topless, in the process of my reconstruction.

"I'm trying to do this as clinically as I can, Pat," whispered Dale with a softness to his voice I hadn't heard before. When I started to cry, he held a scarf to my chest and hugged me. He was uncomfortable too.

"Okay, let's try again," I said emphatically, intent on my mission. Dale with his associate Jaime assisting him, adjusted the lights as I turned various ways. As a little girl, I used to fantasize about posing for a real life photographer when I became a famous model and actress. I never imagined it to be this. But I continued to smile to the camera, occasionally stopping to dab away my tears, and then I'd smile again.

Conflicting emotions drove a horrible headache into me. Though I was deeply touched by the way these two men donated their time to help me document my journey, as a woman I felt mortified. Afterwards, I left with a feeling in the pit of my stomach that wouldn't leave me. Unfortunately, I also left with a little bit of shame.

This is the path I've chosen for my life: to share the story of my cancer with others through the experience of my own breasts. My hope is that through my experience, women will be able to see what this particular breast cancer healing journey and its recovery process *really* looks like. For those going through it, I hope to alleviate some of the fear of the unknown; for the fortunate ones who can still prevent its occurrence, the hope is that they'll be motivated to go for their regular checks-up, be it mammograms, ultrasounds, MRIs, or just a simple self-breast exam. The goal here is to help educate women who have dense breasts but don't know it and to take health into their own hands. A mammogram is not enough! Even sonograms are becoming somewhat obsolete. Be proactive. You can't just accept it; and if they tell you a mammogram is fine and you have dense breasts, you owe it to yourself to find another doctor.

These are a few of the photos from my first photo shoot. They're a bit more G-rated than the second go-round. I would show the second set of photos in private to a breast cancer patient if she wanted to see them.

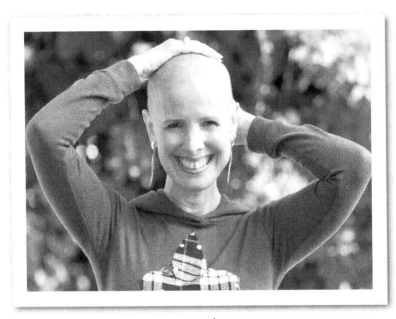

Soft as a baby's tushie

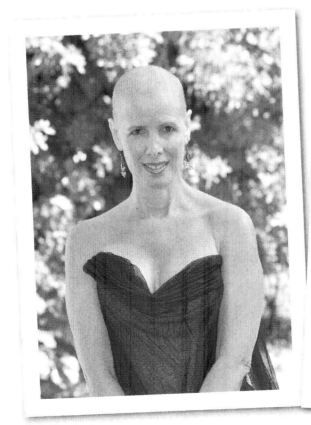

Bald can be sexy

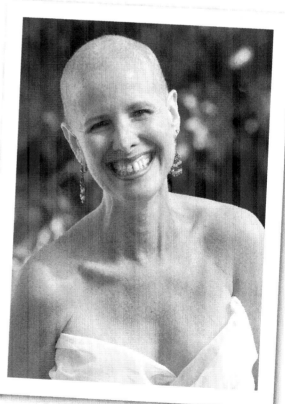

Sometimes you just have to laugh

Christmas was just perfect. Friends and family. Love. Health. Celebrations. I didn't care about my missing nipple anymore. I was a beautiful woman on the inside. The outside would eventually catch up.

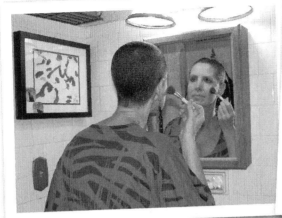

Makeup is a beautiful thing

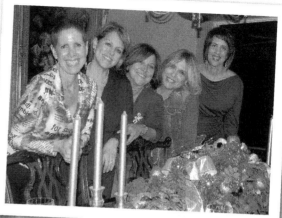

Holiday dinner with my friends

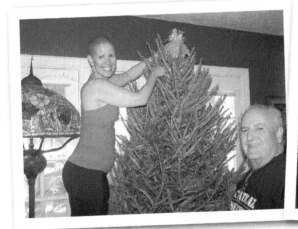

Putting up Xmas tree with my dad

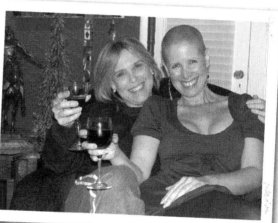

My Angel Annie who cleaned my kitty litter for a year

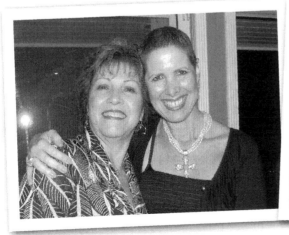

Celebrating with my stepmom

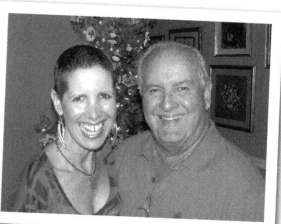

A happy holiday with Papi

The Cancer Dancer

2009

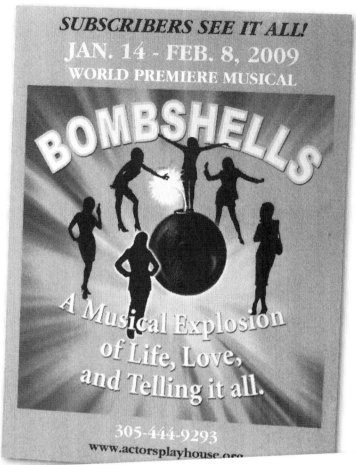

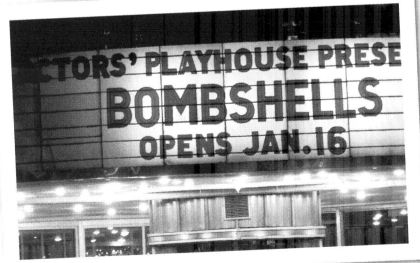

A dream come true

Chapter 16: 2009 – Now WHAT?

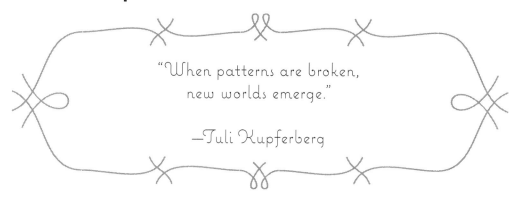

"When patterns are broken,
new worlds emerge."

—Tuli Kupferberg

January was a dream. The book we had written was now a musical and it was premiering in Coral Gables. They added a storyline about my cancer. The amazing playwright, Jeanette Hopkins, thanked me for giving her a great opening and ending to the musical. Of course, she was joking (I think).

We were on a magical carpet ride the entire month of January. We went to the musical almost every night. We signed autographs and met fans. It was one of the most amazing moments of my life. The play got amazing reviews. Cancer was almost a distant dream.

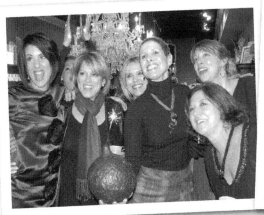

Chocolate Bomb: What a BOMB!

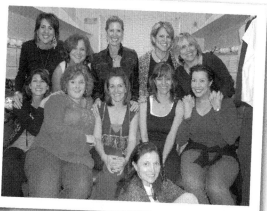

Backstage: Bombshells and
their actor counterparts

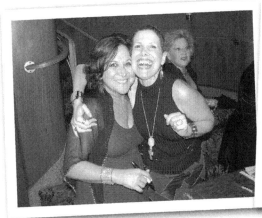

Celebrating with Tammi

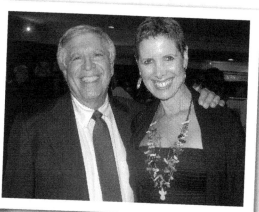

Dr. D comes to Friends and Family Night

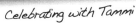

My business had fizzled as I focused on my healing. I was fortunate that I was able to do that, but now ten months later, my mortgage payment was due again and I wasn't sure where the money was going to come from.

I left corporate America and a very hefty salary eight years ago. It was the best decision I had ever made. I was very successful with my company since I had a good reputation for the work that I did. But now, many medical bills later with no clients for the past five months, I was beginning to lose sleep over my lack of income.

Of course, I knew better. I knew that worrying did nothing. Retraining my mind was a daily, pro-active, conscious activity.

I decided to put myself out there. I sent emails to friends and business acquaintances telling them that I was back and ready to work. I looked for full-time employment—that thought made me want to gag a bit, but I had to do something to start paying my bills.

I sent an application to the American Cancer Society® where they had an opening for an assistant director. Now that was something I wouldn't mind doing. I would actually be passionate about that. I just had to trust that things would work out.

Pat's Journal: February 22, 2009

Last night I had the strangest dream. It was a nightmare, actually. I was with a man (I had no idea who this man was), and in the dream we were becoming intimate although he was moving a bit faster than I wanted. He started kissing me, and then suddenly, he reached for my breasts. He then tried to pull my tank top off. I freaked. I had a loose bandage on my left breast, where my newly reconstructed nipple was. As he groped for my breast I screamed, telling him not to take my top off.

I looked down at my breast and it was covered in blood. I woke up horrified and screaming.

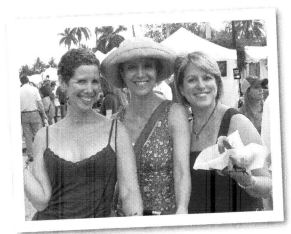

Hitting the Grove Art Festival with my friends

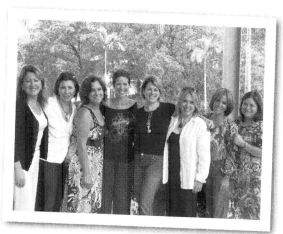

Lunch with girlfriends

I was getting out of the house a lot now. That felt so good. I tried to do as many things as I could outdoors. February in Miami is heavenly.

After worrying one too many days about work, I refocused on dating. I had my first two dates since my breast cancer ordeal. I had two dates in one night. I didn't exactly plan to have two dates in one night, but it just turned out that way. My first date was at 6:30 pm. Drinks. We talked and laughed and enjoyed ourselves. He was sweet and just being out again felt really good. I had a lovely time and by 9:30 pm. I was on my way home.

I received a phone call from a gentleman some friends were trying to set me up with. I was starving, as I had not eaten dinner, so we decided to meet. He was really nice and we had lots of conversation. When I drove myself home, I was ecstatic. I had my mojo back. I was beginning to think my sensuality had gone into hibernation forever. Neither of these guys were the one, but at least I was going out. They seemed to think I was pretty, even with a quarter inch hair.

I felt sexy for the first time in a while. Nine months after my double mastectomy, both thought I was attractive. I was starting to feel normal again. Yep, I was smiling.

Perhaps it was stupid to need outside validation to feel sensual, but as a very female woman, I'm no different than most. I can feel sexy all I want to, but if I don't get attention from a male, especially after having gone through what I just did, it's just not the same.

Last year's birthday gift was certainly an unwanted visitor. This year's birthday surprise was fun and celebratory.

I've always loved birthdays. My friends make fun of me saying that I always turn my birthday into a national holiday. They're probably right. I guess that's what happens when you're an only child and your parents think you're the greatest thing since Cuban sliced bread. I've always had issues with that because I could never live up to those expectations. But the bright side is that my birthdays were always a cause for celebration. And I carried that into adulthood. It was also a great reason to party. And everyone knows I love a good party. I think everyone should celebrate their birthday in a big way.

So of course, my birthday in the midst of my breast cancer journey was going to be special.

My friends told me they were taking me to dinner at a beautiful restaurant on Biscayne Bay.

About 6:00 pm Annie picked me up and told me we were picking up Lydia on the way to the restaurant where the others were meeting us. I was happy to be spending this day with my closest friends even though I was hoping for a party. Starting next year, every birthday would involve parties. I wanted to celebrate and be grateful for every second I was allowed to breathe the air on this beautiful earth.

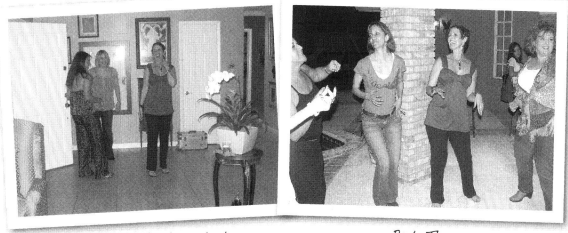

I was REALLY surprised   Party Time

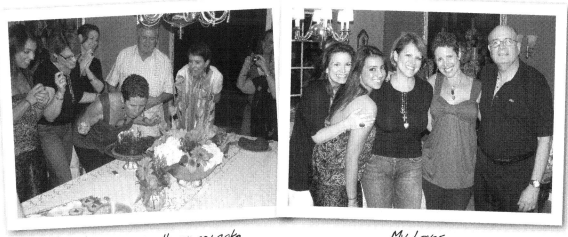

I love every candle on my cake   My Loves

We arrived at Lydia's house. As I walked in, I received the greatest birthday surprise ever. All my family and friends were there. I couldn't believe it when they yelled surprise. I cried. I laughed. I loved it, and I celebrated all night.

Since Santa hadn't brought me both my nipples, I decided that a nipple would be a good birthday gift to myself. Dr. Marshall told me it would be a simple outpatient procedure so Lydia and I headed over with high hopes. We took the video camera and Lydia taped the entire procedure. I couldn't look.

They numbed me locally and then Dr. Marshall got to work. I wasn't looking, but Lydia said Dr. Marshall was meticulously creating art. She centered my left nipple that was a little off to the side and she started building the right nipple, like a cinnamon bun. She twisted the skin until it formed a little ball. She then tattooed my areola, adding more color.

I felt nothing. When it was done, I was bandaged up.

"How did it go?" I asked.

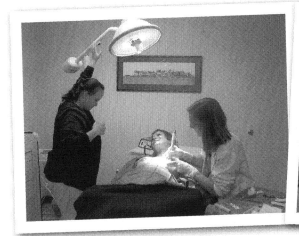

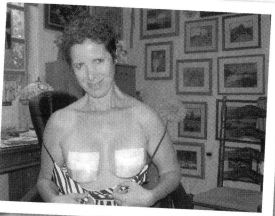

Second nipple surgery   *All bandaged up*

She said, "I was able to build the nipple up just a little, but not completely. The skin was still very tight and I didn't want to tear it."

This wasn't the news I wanted to hear, but I was happy to at least know what to expect. And I agreed. I did not want my skin to rip.

A week later when I took the bandages off, I discovered the tiniest of bumps. My left nipple was perfect. But the right one was challenged. At this point, I didn't really care anymore. I looked good and felt great, although I would never have sensation in my breasts again.

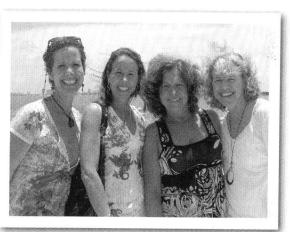

Tammi and her two sisters who had breast cancer, Jodi and Randi

Spending time with friends and family became a priority for me. This cancer had opened my eyes. *Make the time!*

For the first time, my dad and Vivian came with me to a treatment. I had kept them away knowing it would be tough for them. But now I was just on Herceptin® and my dad was more positive. Go figure.

I also started to eat healthier than ever. I learned about juicing greens. This was so not my normal. But neither was cancer. From now on, I would do everything I could to stay healthy. I learned a lot about juicing from Kris Carr. She has great recipes at **www.CrazySexyCancer.com**.

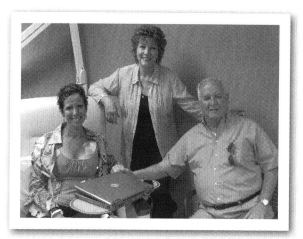

With Papi and Vivian during Herceptin

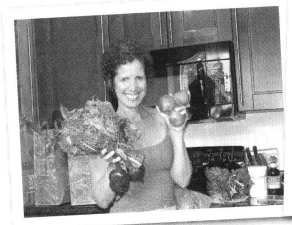

A new way to live and eat

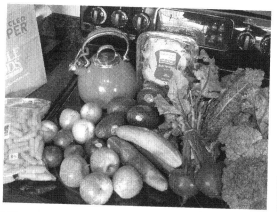

Let the juicing begin

Pat's Journal: June 1, 2009

It's done. My one year of chemo treatment is done. I'm DONE! My archangels Lydia and Tammi were there when the final bell rang. The last bag of Herceptin was empty. Finished! Ding. Ding. Ding. It's done.

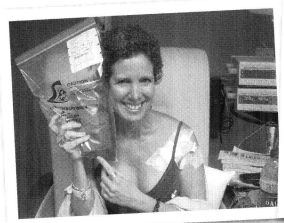

Last bag of sacred juice

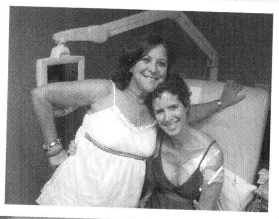

From first chemo to last, Tammi was there

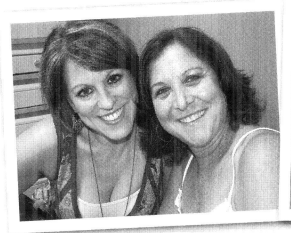

My angels

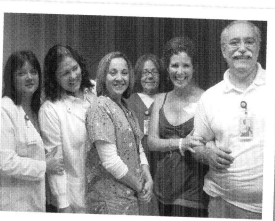

My healers

I can't believe that it's been a whole year. I had 17 sessions of chemo and I swear it doesn't feel like it was that much. Tammi gets upset when I say that it wasn't so hard. She reminds me of those days when I could hardly get out of bed. But truly, it's not what one imagines chemotherapy to be. It's like having a really bad flu sometimes. Sure it isn't a cakewalk, but it's doable.

It was a chance to relax for a year, and a chance to focus on me, my healing, and growth. It's weird, but I feel like it truly was a blessing. It slowed me down. I never spent so much time with the people who matter most in my life. Love surrounded me for an entire year. It's the most amazing and nurturing thing that's ever happened in my life. How bizarre is that? But yes, I'm happy the treatments are finished. Sacred juice—thank you!

Pat's Journal: June 10, 2009

I'm changing the way I live my life. I feel a shift happening. It's strange. It's been a year and two months since my diagnosis. I don't know if it's mental or truly physical, but I'm feeling so much better. I'm exercising now, juicing greens every morning, eating healthier, and meditating more. I'm trying to adjust.

A daily routine that is healthy will be hard for me to do. I just have to remind myself not to get caught up in the daily life and routine of using the blackberry, cell phone, and computer. We all do these things daily and believe we can't live without them. I'm trying to be more aware of my daily life and trying to bring health consciousness into it—physical, emotional, spiritual, and intellectual. I'm feeling really, really good. I'm so excited because I'm getting ready to go on a spiritual journey to Peru—to the sacred mountains that are so healing for me.

My main reason for the trip is to give thanks for my healing. I'm calling it my Gratitude Trip. I have so much to be thankful for. I want to thank God/Spirit; my angels in heaven and on earth; all the medical specialists, doctors, and non-traditional healers; my friends and family; and my medications.

Twenty-five days after my last chemo treatment, I hopped on a plane and headed to Peru with Annie, Kim (another camper I had grown close to), and my sacred stone from Machu Picchu. We were joining my friend Dr. Alberto Villoldo's group from **The Four Winds Shamanic Organization.** Peru was my spiritual home and on this trip I wanted nothing else but to say thank you.

We spent two weeks in the Andes visiting sacred sites and participating in ceremonies in places such as Machu Picchu, Pumamarca, Racchi, Moray, Sacsayhuaman, Tipon, and Pisac. We worked with the Q'eros—shamans who are the descendants of the Inca. We had fire ceremonies at night at 12,000 feet of elevation under the Southern Cross. The life-energy that flowed through me

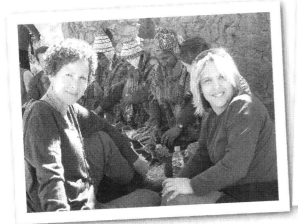

Ceremony of healing and
gratitude with Annie

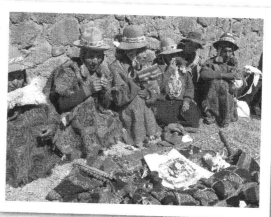

Despacho Ceremony with the Q'ero

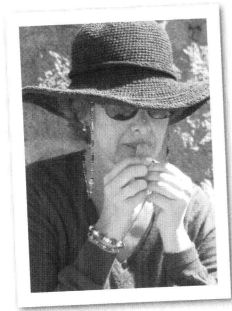

Gratitude prayer

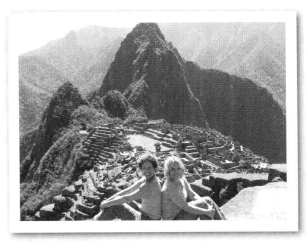

In Machu Picchu

was even greater than I had experienced before. I still had one year of chemo in my body, but I had more energy than most on the trip. I climbed mountains as if floating on air. The magic of the Andes was carrying me up to the very top where I would weep and give thanks.

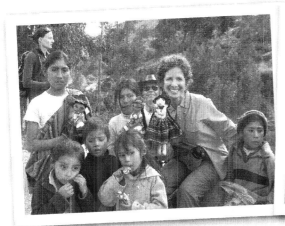

Special moment with local children

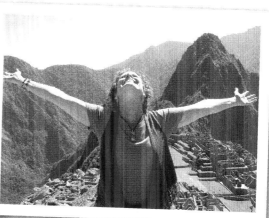

Giving thanks

The Cancer Dancer

2010

Chapter 17: 2010 – Not Without Hope

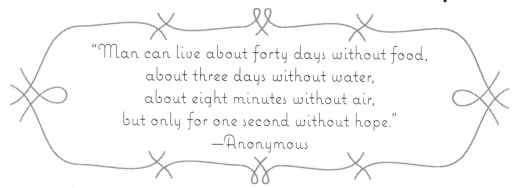

*"Man can live about forty days without food,
about three days without water,
about eight minutes without air,
but only for one second without hope."*
—Anonymous

I still had no idea where I was going with my life. This was the first time I'd ever done this: just threw myself into the hands of God and said, "Okay, do what you want with me. I just hope that I'm able to be happy, healthy, in peace, and loved."

I was determined to share, share, and share. During Breast Cancer Awareness Month, I was again asked to participate in a variety of television and radio shows. I may seem like an extrovert, but those who know me, know that I'm a fraud—I am an introvert pretending to be an extrovert. Public speaking does not come naturally to me.

I was honored and humbled to do what I could do to pay it forward. I did interviews with local TV stations, several radio stations, and was featured in *The Miami Herald's* Breast Cancer Awareness Month special section. My goal was to remind women to get routine exams, to take their health into their own hands, to find out if they have dense breasts and if they did, to get more than just a mammogram—possibly an ultrasound and maybe even an MRI. I had always done what I could during Breast Cancer Awareness Month as a tribute to my mom.

I was invited to be an inspirational keynote speaker at half a dozen major events including Day of Caring, United Way®, Florida International University, and at a pharmaceutical global conference in Lucerne, Switzerland. I spoke in front of 500 people from 40 countries in Switzerland. I never imagined myself as an inspirational speaker.

While I was in Switzerland, I thought, *What did I want to be when I grew up? How would I start a new career at 53? How would I become a public speaker and talk about turning any difficult situation into something positive, when I'm still having a hard time doing that all the time?*

Most of the people I met at this conference were overwhelmed with work and wanting more on the personal side. Everyone seemed to have a problem disconnecting. The corporate life brought some wonderful benefits, namely money, but at what price? How could people and corporations alike begin a new journey?

Much has been written about the work/life balance, but I think it's time to view having a healthy balance of personal time with work as normal. After all, when you're on your deathbed do you really think you'll be reviewing your latest profit and losses before the fat lady sings? Will it be your boss or your corporate board that you want to say your last words to?

I met many people on the trip that lived in one city and their spouse and children lived in another. Sometimes they were 5,000 miles apart. They lived stressful lives. They felt guilty when they were working and not with their family, and guilty when they were with their family and not working. They all knew something wasn't right but weren't quite sure what to do about it. All this for money? Power? I'm not against money or accomplishing goals, but I just worry that we're sacrificing a heck of a lot in order to do that. Both men and women.

I made a decision 30 years ago not to have children. Now, at 53, even though I don't regret that decision, I do feel lonely at times. What would be my legacy? Who would hold me at night and want to hear every single moment of my successes? Who would massage my back and caress my head when sadness struck?

So here I was flying back from Switzerland in the midst of turbulent weather. No one to hold my hand. No one to calm my nerves. So I drank wine and wrote. I prayed that my words would be read by someone. The plane rocked and rolled. I prayed that the winds opened a smooth tunnel for us. And so it did. It just smoothed out as I wrote those words. I thought, *Thank you, sweet God, for my beautiful angels who always come through for me. You know how I love You. And how much faith I have in You.*

The year 2010 continued to be wonderful. I traveled a bit for pleasure. I visited Tammi who had moved to Los Angeles. I started to gain some semblance of normalcy in my life. It was a new normal with less doctor appointments and more time for me away from the medical world. I didn't journal much. Perhaps I needed a break.

But a few big things happened that year. Life introduced me to a new type of dance partner— wonderful women streaming into my life from all different directions. My doctors and nurses called on me to help patients who needed a shot of positivity, encouragement, and guidance. Their trust in me was part of what fueled my passion to be of service to those in need. People called after hearing me on television and radio shows. Friends and strangers referred women to me. They were all breast cancer patients looking for the same things: information, inspiration, and hope. I became a patient advocate, paying it forward.

Simultaneously, I struggled to make a living. Yet, I couldn't stop myself from spending my days helping these strong, shining women. It's pro bono. I'm not getting paid to do this. But what does it matter? Money will not make their scars go away. Money will not take their fear away. The more women I met, the more I realized that we were all part of a sisterhood and it was our duty to help one another on this journey. So, I started to bring together women on a monthly basis that were going through/or had gone through breast cancer. We called ourselves The Link of Hope Sistas. We encouraged, inspired, and educated each other. They were all beautiful and courageous and dealing with the roller coaster that is life and cancer. We met monthly at my home. We were Sistas and that bond would never be broken.

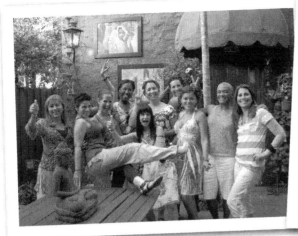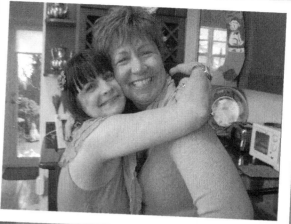

Fun with my beautiful Link of Hope Sistas   Friendships developed quickly: Cindy hugging on Debbie

Debbie Cabrera, one of the Sistas, said this about our group:

> The **Link of Hope** is a true blessing sent from a higher source. Whatever you need to know is revealed to you exactly when you need it. The Sistas have been my "go-to" place, my source of information. We are a multi-cultural, highly skilled group of professional women with no filters: you ask, the group shares. There are solid references for doctors, nutrition, treatments, and information on ways to deal with side effects.
>
> I could compare and contrast. It was key in maintaining my spiritual balance. After speaking to them, I felt that I was able to tackle this opportunity with no problem at all. They enabled both my daughter and me to share with others that are starting on this journey. We must have faith in order to be healed. Never believe in limitations. I love my Sistas.

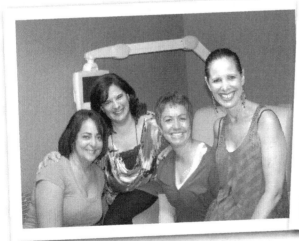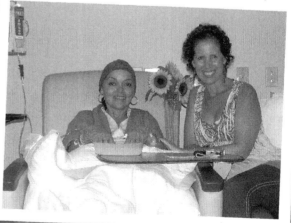

Link of Hope Sista Debbie's first chemo   Link of Hope Sista Elena in chemo

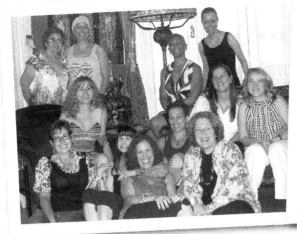

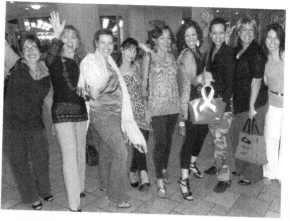

Silly Sista fun   *Out on the town with the Sistas*

I was committed, through speaking engagements and through my Sistas, to take the message of hope around the world. I desired to encourage others to stay positive when times were tough, to live life to the fullest no matter what comes their way, and to remember that the sun is always shining behind the clouds.

This was also the year that I started to look like myself again. My hair was growing out and my breasts were looking pretty good. This disease really played havoc with my vanity. It had a unique way of making me feel less feminine. My cancer hit me right where it hurt—at the core of my womanhood and sensuality. I had a constant struggle with self-esteem but I was beginning to feel good about myself again.

And then it happened. "Mr. Right" showed up at Books & Books. On July 9, 2010, I met Patricio. He was a beautiful man, inside and out. It was like I had traveled full-circle. I received the "you have cancer" call in this same book store and now Mr. Right was standing in front of me.

From the moment we met, I felt like we'd known each other forever. He was really, really handsome. But as we talked, I could tell that he was humble and sweet, kind and compassionate. He loved animals, was fluent in English, Spanish, and French, and born in Chile. He was open to learning more about spirituality and he danced!

Patricio writes:

> *When I first saw Pat I was immediately captivated by her beauty. We met at Books & Books in Coral Gables. When our eyes met for the first time, we both smiled. It was like we knew this was something special. We made some small talk. We checked each other out in our own subtle ways. I think we both liked what we saw and how we felt. It was so funny that she was Patricia and I was Patricio. Hmm . . . meant to be?*

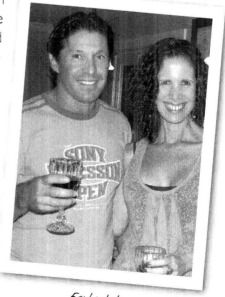

Early date

We chatted for a little bit then decided to take it a step further and go to dinner. I invited her to my favorite Japanese restaurant down the street that happened to be her favorite, too. A coincidence?

We walked the few blocks while stealing glances at each other, checking each other out. We were like two teenagers. Our smiles could barely fit on the sidewalk. We were engorged with this deliciously uncontrollable attraction. Pat taught me that night to drink hot sake followed by a sip of cold beer. I usually did not drink much but when I did, I drank it like water. Pat pointed out, "It's not that you don't drink, you just don't drink well."

Luckily I did keep my composure and remained sober. We had a wonderful dinner. Her smiley eyes made it easy for me to feel comfortable. As the evening progressed, I realized I was in the presence of someone special. It wasn't so much what she said. There was a certain aura about her that gave her an almost angelical demeanor. She gave me the impression that she was at peace with herself. She was very sure of herself but her expression was humble and compassionate. Her smile was so sweet and honest. After dinner it was obvious that we didn't want to end our evening yet. We walked side-by-side to a nearby café. We sat at a corner table and had a cup of decaf coffee. We talked while a cellist played beautiful Latin favorites in another room. It was another magical moment in our wonderful evening.

Our evening didn't quite end there. Pat confessed to me that one of her passions was dancing. I think that I was put through a series of tests that night without my knowledge. Dancing was the last test of the evening. We found a nearby night club where they played Latin music.

She guided me through the salsa and said she liked the way I danced. I think I was "approved"! At about 2:00 am our evening came to an end. I walked her to her car. We felt a sweet closeness—we were two souls that didn't know each other a few hours ago and now we were face-to-face with our first good night. A quick kiss and a long glance sealed the night.

The following evening, I invited her to attend a wedding with me. We had an amazing night and we already felt like we were boyfriend and girlfriend.

Walking hand-in-hand after the soccer World Cup finals the next day, Pat stopped suddenly and said "I have something I really need to tell you. I had breast cancer two years ago. I had a double mastectomy, one year of chemo, reconstruction . . . and I'm okay. But you need to know this."

I think I reacted as if I already knew about it. I don't know why, but something told me she had gone through a major life challenge and won. When she said this to me, my heart totally opened up. She was right. It had been a blessing—for her and now for me. She said that this had been the best thing that had ever happened to her. I could not expect anything other than such a response from her. It all fit perfectly. Pat's attitude in the face of what would be a tragedy for most is testimony of her fortitude. She explained that her cancer was simply an uninvited guest in her body. This guest had the purpose to bring her awareness and growth. I don't know why or how, but I understood exactly what she meant.

I was falling madly in love with Patricia San Pedro. Or, as she liked to correct me, "You are falling sanely in love."

I love everything about her. The fact that she had breast cancer just makes her more beautiful to me. I wouldn't change a thing about her. This was when we were supposed to come into each other's life. I was supposed to love her in her newly acquired beauty. In my eyes there was no one that could surpass her beauty. She said that I see her with eyes of love. As if those eyes were not real. Of course I saw my woman through the lens of love. How else would I see her? On one of her videos that Pat recorded during her healing journey, she asked the question, "Would I ever be sexy again?"

Under the circumstances, in the midst of her chemo, I could understand why she would have those doubts. But to me, there was no doubt. She WAS sexy. Her radiant beauty went beyond her physical attributes. There was an aura of peace about her that made her even lovelier. Yes, this was when I was supposed to come into her life. I was forever the luckiest man.

Our journey together has just begun. It promises to be a journey of love, healing, and growth. One of Pat's doorways opened up before her the day she was diagnosed with cancer, revealing countless opportunities to help others. Not only did she not turn away from it, but she has embraced it as a life mission. Now I stand proudly by her side reaffirming my love and support for her and her tireless cause to help others who are affected by cancer.

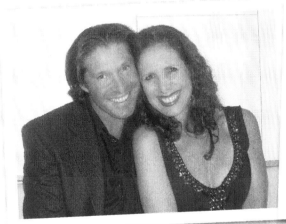

Patricio and Patricia

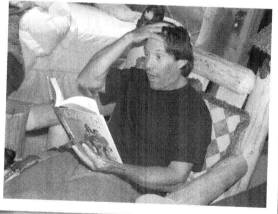

Patricio reads my book for the first time-YIKES!

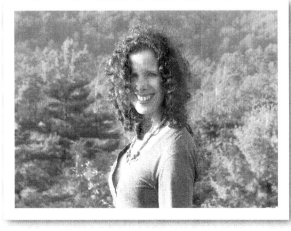

Happy in nature

The Cancer
Dancer

2011

Chapter 18: 2011 – New Morning

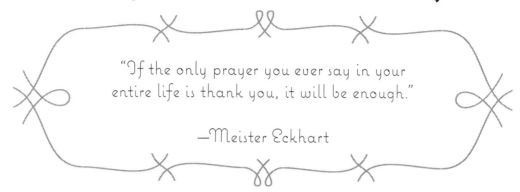

> *"If the only prayer you ever say in your entire life is thank you, it will be enough."*
>
> —Meister Eckhart

I went with Patricio to his homeland of Chile. It was a trip to meet "the family" but also to explore his beautiful roots. I loved every moment of the trip as our love continued to grow. He wasn't with me on my healing journey, but he was here now, when I needed him most.

I was scheduled for my three-month check up with Dr. Glück two months after our return from Chile. The morning began like most others. I was still tired after a night of insomnia. I guess that's what happened at the age of post-menopause, post-chemo, and an over-active mind.

In my deepest of deepest places I knew that I was healed and cancer-free. Yet there was always this tiny speck of worry, when you go for that face-to-face encounter with your doctor.

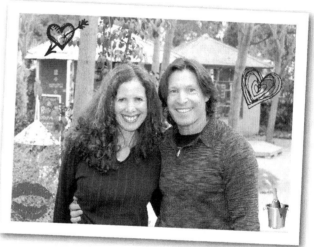

Patricio and me in Chile

Patricio came with me. As we entered Sylvester Comprehensive Cancer Center, the familiar signs and smells came back to me. It wasn't until I walked through its halls that my cancer journey confronted the center of my consciousness.

It was wonderful to see all the nurses. These healing angels poured love, kindness, and compassion into all of their patients. They made me feel like I was the most special of them all. I'm sure every patient felt the same way. And what a gift that was. How great it was to feel illuminated.

This was the first time that Patricio came to one of my doctor appointments. I gave him a complete color-commentary of the building, the nurses, and the procedures: it did my heart good to share this with him. It was the first time I came here without my angels in tow. This time, I had Patricio.

The sweet nurses that work with Dr. Glück, Odalys, and Jennifer, took their time with me going over my chart. They checked my blood pressure and examined me. It all looked good. When they left, Dr. Glück arrived. We talked as he checked under my arms, around my breasts, and under the neck.

"All looks great," he said. "You're all clear. Done. You don't have to return until next year."
I was somewhat confused. "What do you mean?" I asked.

"You're done. You are cancer-free. It's been three years. That's it."

I said, "I thought it wasn't until five years that you got the 'all-clear.'"

"It depends on the type of cancer. You are estrogen-negative, so the mark is three years for you."

I couldn't believe it. I think I was somewhat in shock. I wasn't expecting this news for another two years. What do you mean? I'll just come back once a year? A part of me felt somewhat relieved while the other side felt a bit rejected. I know that sounded weird, but these check-ups had been a constant in my life for the past three years.

I walked out somewhat numb. I took Patricio on a tour of the chemo area. I wanted to say hi to all the wonderful nurses that gave me my chemotherapy for a year. They were as thrilled to see me as I was to see them. They couldn't believe my hair. Yep, it was back in full force. I thanked each one of them for my healing. They were angels from above.

As we waited for the valet to bring our car around, the emotions started to come up. I thought I was going to explode into tears right there in front of everyone. Tears came up to my eyes as I put on my sunglasses. My throat tightened. I rushed into the car as Patricio turned to hug me and whispered, "Congratulations."

I broke down. There were so many emotions, so many memories. I was so grateful; so very, very, very grateful.

I was cancer-free. I was totally healed and healthy. Oh glorious day. I couldn't wait to tell everyone.

I called Lydia, Maria, and Tammi. They were ecstatic, as I knew they would be. Then I called my dad and stepmom.

I said, "I have a surprise to share with both of you." They held their breath, thinking that I was going to tell them I eloped. "I am cancer-free," I announced. "I got the all-clear."

I could not have had the strength to survive if it wasn't for my mother. My mom infused in me her extraordinary strength, spirit, and positivity so that I never saw breast cancer as anything other than something that would make me a better person.

I am grateful for my life, my healing, and the angels who carried me on their wings. I am grateful for the amazing dance with cancer that changed my life forever.

Now I state loudly and affirmatively THANK YOU. I do my best to live life in balance. I eat healthy and am trying to exercise regularly. I meditate and connect with Spirit. I'm helping others and living my life on purpose. I affirm. I am happy. I am healthy. I am joyful. I am calm. I am. I am. I am.

Cancer slowed me down, taking me off the fast-track and placing me on a gentler course. Now, I let life take the lead. I am learning to dance a new dance . . . one step at a time.

The Cancer Dancer

Patient-to-Patient
and Caregiver Tips

Week One: The Diagnosis

You've just had a biopsy. The waiting begins and the waiting time period may vary. For instance, my doctor called me the next day, but I have friends who waited a week which was pure agony. Always ask your doctor how long lab results will take and push for a quick turnaround.

Next you have to determine if you want to be by yourself or have someone by your side when you get your results. I knew I didn't want to be alone when the call came with the biopsy results. I wanted and needed to be with someone I loved and who loved me back. Your doctor may want to give you the news in person, or you might get a phone call like I did. So think about who you want with you, if anyone. You might hear life-changing news.

However, if you are reading this, you have probably heard that dreaded word. Please, **don't** equate cancer with death. Just because D follows C in the alphabet, one does not have to follow the other! Yes, the news will rock your world, and you may start to feel it is crumbling around you. Stop. Breathe. And start to build your own house of faith and positivity, brick by brick, because *that* is what will determine how you heal.

Start keeping a record of all your appointments. Actually, have an official record-keeper. You won't remember anything. Assign this to one of your most reliable friends/family members.

Follow-up Radiologist Visit

After you get the news, you'll go to see the radiologist again. Take a loved one with you.

Ask him/her to take notes. You will not remember a thing when you walk out. These notes are critical. Make sure to bring in a list of questions that you write down beforehand. The both of you should ask as many questions as possible. The Susan G. Komen website has good downloadable questions that you can take with you. **http://ww5.komen.org/**

Take what the doctor says seriously. But only God/Spirit knows what is in store for you. Once again, keep your faith and a positive outlook.

Ask your radiologist for recommendations. Who is the best breast surgical oncologist they know? Who is the best oncologist? Ask them to make an appointment for you right then and there. My radiologist, Dr. Biaggi, picked up the phone and scheduled me with the best of the best, Dr. Robert DerHagopian, for three days later.

Be lovingly aggressive in getting what you need.

Ask for information that you can read on your own. However, for me I decided to not go over the top on reading material. It can be overwhelming.

I made a decision early not to read all the "bad stuff" out there. You'll always find depressing information, either prognosis statistics or news on terrible side effects from drugs. Blah, blah,

blah. I wasn't in denial, but I truly wanted to serve myself a daily requirement of news that would heal and serve me. My friends did a lot of the research on their own. They became just as educated on the subject of breast cancer. But if someone started to give me "downer" information, I stopped them. Thanks, but no thanks. I'm healing. End of conversation.

I educated myself online, by speaking with survivors and talking with professionals in the medical profession that I trust. My friend Sally Bogert, an oncology nurse who has worked in research, educated me to the point of knowing what to expect from the surgeon on Monday and some of the specific questions to ask. However, I did not overwhelm myself with information and I especially did not dwell on all the possible negative side effects. I focused on education and positive outcomes.

Week Two: Surgical Visit

First, you should ask around and get to the very best breast surgical oncologist possible.

Once again, you will want to take a loved one with you. They need to take notes and ask the right questions.

Lydia and Tammi bought me a beautiful leather-bound journal. I filled it with my own notes, questions, feelings and anything else that made me happy. Tammi and Lydia each had their own notebooks that they carried throughout my entire healing journey.

You might want to consider journaling. Chronicling my way through illness has saved me. It has also given me time to express who I am rather than how my illness defined me. Journaling or chronicling your cancer can be an opportunity to have a better relationship with yourself and experience your cancer in all its stages (good, bad, and yucky). Journal, video and ask your friends to keep their own journals based on their own perspectives of your cancer. This will be a life-changing experience for everyone.

Prepare for your visit to the surgeon, once again with a list of good questions. As I mentioned before, the Susan G. Komen website has good downloadable questions that you can take with you. http://ww5.komen.org/

Suggestions for your first meeting with the surgeon

- My friend Tammi says to bake a Bundt® cake to every doctor's visit. The doctor and staff will love you even more.

- Find out what ALL your options are. Only YOU can decide what's best for you.

- Move quickly. The doctor might be wonderful, but it's your body. You want the cancer out ASAP. So insist on having all the necessary tests done within the next week and set up a date and time for your surgery.

- You are your own best health advocate. Don't be shy. It's your life we're talking about here.

Insist on having a **BRCA Genetic Test** before your surgery. The BRCA Genetic Test is a blood test that uses DNA analysis to identify harmful changes (mutations) in either one of the two breast cancer susceptibility genes—BRCA1 and BRCA2. Women who have inherited mutations in these genes face a much higher risk of developing breast cancer and ovarian cancer compared with the general population. I know a lady who was not tested prior to her lumpectomy. She went through chemo and radiation. Several years later her cancer returned. This time she was tested. Turns out she was BRCA positive. Had she had the test the first time around, she would have had both breasts and her ovaries removed right then and there. The tough part about this is getting your insurance to cover it. Be persistent. If you have at least two cases of breast cancer in your close family (even distant family), you're more likely to be covered.

Nurse Navigator

A nurse navigator helps steer cancer patients through the medical system maze. Check with the hospital to see if they provide this service. They are your personal assistants throughout this journey, free of charge.

Nurse navigators walk you through the diagnosis again, answering any questions. They help you understand your diagnosis, overcome any fears, and provide access to your medical records and treating physicians. They also can be an interface on insurance issues.

They help you schedule your oncology, surgery, and radiation appointments. They work around your work schedule, can accompany you to any or all of your appointments, and can wait for you when you come out of recovery. They are angelic. Sometimes, you don't even have to talk. They just know.

Breast Reconstruction

Educate yourself on all the options for breast reconstruction. There are many: some have been around for years and some are breakthrough. There are implants, which is what I have. There is a variety of flap procedures available. And then there is a new breakthrough procedure coming out of Miami. Dr. Roger Khouri at the Miami Breast Center rebuilds an entire breast from fat. It's never been done this particular way before. There is no cutting, no incisions, no scars, no implants, no flaps, and no major surgery. It's amazing. *AND* women keep sensation in their breasts, which is something I'll never have. In the past women who wanted breasts with their own fat had to undergo eight hour flap procedures and they're numb in the end. No more!

Since I was not aware of Dr. Khouri's procedure at the time of my surgery, I went for the implants. I am very happy with my new girls although I would have opted for Dr. Khouri's procedure had I known about it. Dr. Dierdre Marshall did an amazing job for me. I still have only one nipple, but that's due to the fact that I have very thin skin where the cancer was and building another nipple there might tear the skin. So, I'll live as a "nipple Cyclops" my entire life. I really don't care. Neither does my boyfriend.

You'll want your reconstruction plastic surgeon right there when you have your mastectomy. Once your surgical oncologist is done, the plastic surgeon comes in.

Sacred Spaces and Healing Things

Feed your spirit and connect. Now's the time to put your faith into practice if you haven't already done so. I've always been spiritual, but I shifted into high gear when I was diagnosed.

I'm sharing some of the things that worked for me. Of course, do whatever brings you peace, comfort, and a connection to Spirit so you can heal from the inside out.

Make time for your spiritual connection—at least one hour per day.

Create a sacred space in your home. I have a little corner in my bedroom. In my space I have things that are sacred and comforting to me:

- Inspirational music. (I loved the *Soulfood* CD Sky Spirit; all of Carlos Nakai's music; the heali song "I am Holy" by Here II Here and Jack Kassewitz, **www.hereiihere.com**)

- Sage

- Soy candles

- Cushions to sit on for meditation

- Sacred stones and other sacred objects

- Journal/books (with affirmations, meditations, and uplifting messages)

- Angel cards

- Chakra tuning bell

Meditate. Pray. Connect with Spirit. God. The Universe. Whomever/whatever you believe in. I believe it will help you on your healing journey. I know it's helped me on mine. Don't know how to meditate? Here are a few tips:

- Turn off all the phones.

- Tell others in your home that you're in private time.

- Make sure you're in a quiet place where you can just go and meditate.

- You can meditate for five minutes up to an hour, whatever works for you. No rules here. For me, 20 minutes in the morning and 20 minutes at night were wonderful. It brought me tremendous peace, centering, and healing. It stopped my brain from going in many directions.

- Meditating is just sitting in a quiet position. I do what works for me. I hold onto my stones and I just close my eyes and take a deep breath for the first few seconds. Then I just sit in silence. When thoughts come my way, I push them aside and place them on a shelf. I don't judge them. I will deal with them later. I just sit in silence and connect. There's a beauty and peace and a tranquility that comes with that and when the day gets crazy, somehow you're able to tap into the silence and the peace if you do this regularly.

Breast MRI

Once again, if possible, have someone take you. It always calmed my nerves to have a loved one with me.

Stretch before the MRI. Stretch your arms and neck. You want to be flexible because you'll be holding a non-moving position for a while.

Before you go in, ask your technician to count you down. It helped me to know when we had ten minutes left, five minutes left, and so on.

MRI machines are *VERY* loud—annoyingly loud actually. Remember that so you won't be surprised.

Close your eyes and relax as best you can. It's not comfortable because you'll lay face down with your breasts through two holes and your forehead lands on hard plastic. I have no idea why they don't cushion that plastic frame, but they don't.

Bring your own soothing music to MRI and Pet Scans.

Now this might seem strange to you, but I pretended that the very loud thudding noises coming from the machine were Indian drums. I used the sound to help me meditate and take myself to a different place. I envisioned the lights and sounds being healing, taking me to a relaxed place of health and peace.

PET Scan

Bring along your favorite CD or music that will help you relax. Once again, have someone take you. They can bring a book while they wait.

First, they will inject dye into your veins and you just hang out for an hour or so. You can't do anything, so just sleep, meditate, or relax.

Once you go into the PET Scan room, give them your CD with music to relax you. I had Native American flute music—my favorite kind. They will play it for you while you're having the scan.

I envisioned the lights and sounds that came from the equipment to be healing. I used them to put me in a bit of a trance state so that I remained relaxed. Together with my music, it really calmed me down. It worked!

Living Your New Life During Treatment

Have Positive Thoughts Only!

- Start to learn the lessons you need to learn from this experience and receive all the blessings. There are many.

- If people around you are negative; send them away with love.

- Stay away from the news. You don't need anything depressing in your radar. Focus on your healing and that's it.

- If situations around you are toxic, stay clear of them.

- Let others deal with problems and daily life.

- Release control: If they don't do it "your way," it's okay. The world will keep spinning. I guarantee it.

- Spend time with people who nurture you.

- Don't let others take you into conversations that are not healing.

- Read uplifting books. Stay away from drama on television, in books, and in your daily life, too.

- End your day with a gratitude prayer with five things you're grateful for.

Caregivers Tips

When someone hears the words "You have cancer," it is a diagnosis for the entire family and the closest of friends. You will all travel this healing journey together and it can be a beautiful time to bond, heal and discovery new blessings in your life, if you make the decision to do so.

Below are a few tips for the caregivers/families/friends

What NOT to Say

A few people have come up to me and said things like, "Ooooooh breast cancer? Oh no! My mother-in-law died of breast cancer." Can you imagine? So I look at them like . . . um . . . okay. I think maybe people just freeze and don't know what to say. So if someone tells you they have breast cancer, don't say you know someone who died from it!

Caregivers Tips Cont'd

What To Do:

- Be with her, even if she says she wants to be alone. At least that's my own personal belief. Support her in any and every way possible. Of course, there are times she will need alone time. It's a contradiction, I know. Just trust your heart.

- Cook for her, clean for her, and sit with her even if she's napping while you sit in her living room and read.

- Help her create a sacred healing space and a positive attitude.

- Don't bring her down. Don't look at it as something horrendous that's happening to her. Accept the fact that this is her path and then be her support. This isn't about you. It's about her.

- Give her love. Nurture her.

- Do not pity her. It's not healthy for the recovery process.

- Allow her to have "bad days." There will be days when she is moody or snaps easily. Be patient and remind yourself of what she is going through.

- Remember you are human and what is happening is affecting you, too. Make time for yourself. Give yourself your space and find things to do on your own to clear your head. If you're not at peace with yourself, you will not be capable of helping your loved one.

- When she feels up for it, let her handle chores and run errands to help you out. It lets her feel productive and needed.

- Have a sense of humor.

- Include her in your life. Talk to her about what's going on in your life, your work, and your plans for the future. Keep her in the loop.

- Do fun things together. Play games and watch movies. Enjoy life together!

- Whenever possible, accompany her to doctor's appointments. Become involved, ask questions and develop a rapport with the doctor. It shows your support to both your relative/friend and her doctor.

- Keep a positive attitude. It's contagious.

Pre-Mastectomy/Lumpectomy:

Pre-op Shopping list and the reasons why

Prepare for surgery by going shopping. Here is a list that will be very helpful.

☐ Comfy slippers for the hospital.

☐ Clothing that you can easily get in and out of when you can't raise your arm(s) after a mastectomy or lumpectomy. Have buttons on the front of everything: pajamas, shirts, dresses. All of it. Buy large sizes for comfort and buy clothing with soft material so it won't be uncomfortable resting near your stitches.

☐ Robe with simple wrap belt at the waist so you can adjust as needed. You can also look into the Velcro robes. Make sure your robe is lightweight. It just feels better than walking around the hospital in its "designer" robe.

☐ Silky pajamas. The silk will feel soft against your skin.

☐ Eye mask and ear plugs or headphones. Nurses are in all day and night so if you have your eyes and ears covered, you may be able to get a bit of sleep.

☐ Bulky or heavy stuff that you will need later (paper towels, toilet paper, dog/cat food, drinks) so you don't have to worry about that after surgery.

☐ Travel pillow. It is the best for resting your head and arms in the hospital and at home after surgery.

☐ Seat belt shoulder pad for cushioning the seatbelt in your car.

☐ Large safety pins (to attach drains to your clothing).

☐ Pants with pockets (to put drains in when you don't want to pin them to blouses). Get only pull-on pants. Zippers and snaps are difficult to manage.

☐ Sweatpants. *Be comfortable:* that's my motto.

☐ Wash cloths for the shower.

☐ Hemorrhoid pads (Tucks®). You'll use them to clean your arm pits when you get home so you don't smell. You won't be able to shower for at least 10 days after surgery and you don't want to be smelly.

☐ Journal and maybe a video camera if you decide to document your journey.

☐ Soothing music for your room so you can hear it after surgery. I brought my Native American flute music to the surgery itself. Had them play it IN surgery! The nurses and doctors loved it too.

☐ Nursing pads: they sell them everywhere; they will cushion your breasts

☐ Roomba® Cleaning Robot: this vacuum cleans by itself; I highly recommend it

☐ Electric razor: you won't have feeling under your arm and you do not want to cut yourself

☐ Electric toothbrush (easier to brush)

☐ Plastic cups and straws for home: lighter and easier to lift than glass, and no cleanup (it's not great for the environment but it's just for a few weeks)

☐ Books, magazines, DVDs

☐ Hand-held shower so someone can shampoo your hair at home easily

☐ Long-handled hair brush (easier to brush)

☐ Dog/cat food and treats: your little ones will not leave your side and they will help you heal

☐ Healthy drinks in the event you don't feel like eating (anesthesia made my stomach yucky for a few days)

☐ Lots of pillows: you'll want them all over the house for support

☐ Prunes and stool softeners at home (pain meds are constipating)

☐ Lip balm

☐ Soft cami tops: you'll start to wear them a few days after surgery (buy the ones with the shelf bras in them)

☐ Body lotion to make you feel and smell girly

☐ Saline eye drops

☐ A comfy Lazy Boy®-type chair to sleep and sit in during the day: it's way easier when you first get home from the hospital to sleep in this, plus it's a great chair to get in and out of with little or no help

Miscellaneous Things To Do Before Your Surgery

☐ Cut your hair so it's easier to manage.

☐ Take pretty pictures of your boobies before your surgery. There's no rewinding that tape.

☐ Create your circle of angels. You have no idea how important this is. Don't be shy. I had about 20 of them. These girlfriends did everything for me. EVERYTHING! Your friends and family will want to help. Tell them NOT to wait for you to ask. Tell them that you need them now and then count on them. And then LET THEM HELP!

My friend Tammi created a calendar and each friend took turns doing things for me—grocery shopping, walking my dog, cleaning the kitty litter, etc. It was a joy to spend so much time with my girlfriends. Even if you have a husband, assign girlfriends to be your angels too.

☐ If you don't have the support system, go in search of a support group. Every community has them.

☐ Connect with someone who has gone through this before. Their advice and support is invaluable. Positively Pat and Link of Hope Sistas are here for you. Connect with us through **www.PositivelyPat.com**. There are many other groups that can help you connect with your own angels/mentors. Here are two: **www.imermanangels.org** and **www.lotussurvivalfoundation.org**.

☐ Don't shave within two days before your surgery or it will increase your risk of infection.

☐ Set up a website on either **www.Carepages.com** or **www.caringbridge.org**. It is super-easy and FREE! It's much easier than having to update people on your progress (which can become exhausting). You have an online journal and the best part is that everyone can sign your guestbook and leave messages.

☐ Set up an "out-of-office" message on your phone/computer so that people at work will know to leave you alone. You need time off to heal.

Stay positive, eat healthy before and after the operation, and rest as much as possible.

The Last Appointment With Your Surgeon Prior To Surgery

☐ Ask him/her to schedule massages (through physical therapy) in the hospital to help with neck and back pain.

☐ Tell your doctor that you want him/her to order a visiting nurse to come and change your drains every day at home (if your insurance will pay for it). It is not necessary, but I found it comforting.

☐ Be sure to ask your plastic surgeon EXACTLY what you are allowed to do after surgery. My surgeon did not want any arm movement or as little as possible until the drains came out about 10 days later. I couldn't write thank you notes or type on the computer since my elbows had to be by my side. I could brush my teeth and eat but that is about all she wanted me to do.

☐ Get your port during your surgery if possible. Why have an extra surgery just for the port? If you have little or thin veins, get a port. My suggestion is to get it in your chest NOT your arm. The port in my arm touched my median nerve and I was in excruciating pain. Eventually, I had to have it moved to my chest.

☐ If you like a private room, ask your surgeon to order it. I am told if the doctor orders it, insurance will cover the expense. If you request it, you'll be billed the difference.

☐ Tell your doctor to order that you stay at least two nights in the hospital. If the doctor orders it, the insurance will pay for it. Otherwise, they send you home within 24 hours which is ridiculous!

☐ Make sure your doctor has left a written prescription for nausea. Most patients coming out of anesthesia have nausea and you don't want to wait around until they find your doctor. Tell them you want the IV form, not oral. When you're nauseated, the last thing you want is a pill.

☐ Discuss lymphedema with your surgeon and ask him/her to measure your arms before and after surgery. Depending on several factors, you might need to wear a compression sleeve after surgery.

A Note On Lymphedema

Lymphedema is the swelling of the arm and quadrant (upper chest and back) where surgery was performed, in which lymph nodes were removed in an effort to stop cancer cells from spreading.

Lymphedema occurs in more than eight percent of women after their surgery, and that number increases to 35 percent in women who have radiation treatment following surgery. Lymphedema in most cases happens right after surgery, but it can even begin up to 30 years later. This is different for everyone. That is why it's important to know the indications, care, and precautions of Lymphedema to understand your risk level.

The most important factor in protecting yourself from lymphedema is recognizing it early. How? If you just had surgery, ask your doctor how many lymph nodes were removed. This will help you determine if you are at a low, medium, or high risk. Remember this only means that you need to be more aware of it, but it still shouldn't alarm you since you will be taking control!

We all have an average of 25 to 30 axillary lymph nodes in each axilla (underarm), and so the greater the number removed, the more awareness to the precautions you will need to take. If radiation is part of your treatment, the intensity and areas radiated will also be a determining factor. Ask your doctor if you are at risk for lymphedema. He or she should be able to answer your questions and concerns and refer you to a lymphedema therapist as needed.

An oncologist told a friend that he could not stress enough to continue physical therapy for her lymphedema even after her treatment was over. Continue wearing the sleeve. He said he had two patients that stopped wearing the sleeve for a year and the arm swelled up completely.

This information was provided by my friend, Ana Maria Mendieta, MSPT, CLT-LANA. She is founder of the Midas Touch Institute, a "one-on-one" physical therapy clinic specializing in the treatment of lymphedema and the Lymphedema Foundation of South Florida (LFSF), a non-profit organization, to help uninsured or underinsured women and men in need of lymphedema therapy treatments. **www.midastouchinstitute.com**

Prepare Your Home Before Your Surgery

☐ In the kitchen, move things you use frequently to lower levels so you can reach them without having to raise your arm(s).

☐ Divide food items into small containers. For example, if you have a gallon of milk, divide it up into four small containers. You won't be able to pick up any weight.

☐ Stay with someone if you live alone or have someone stay with you for at least 10 days.

☐ Set up a phone near the bed/chair you will sit in or keep your cell in your pocket.

☐ Use your speaker phone on your cell. Holding the phone up will be difficult.

☐ Cook and freeze foods prior to surgery.

☐ Pre-pay bills. I knew my brain would be fried and I did not want to think.

☐ If you have a yard or garden, arrange for someone to take care of it.

☐ Set up a chair outside for the times you feel up to sitting outside.

Pre-Op Hospital Visit

☐ Bring a list of all the medications and supplements you are taking before going to the hospital. Otherwise, if you're like me, you'll forget.

In The Hospital

☐ Someone has to sleep with you in the hospital BOTH NIGHTS. Plan it beforehand.

☐ Remind your doctor to get you massages (through physical therapy) in the hospital to help with neck and back pain after surgery.

☐ Use the travel pillow you bought.

☐ Make sure your pain meds are scheduled and not on an as-needed basis. Stress that point with your surgeon and anesthesiologist.

☐ Fill pain meds prescriptions BEFORE leaving the hospital. Ask for that last shot just prior to discharge.

☐ For the ride home, take that seat belt cushion you bought.

I love this tip from a survivor.

"I remember after my first surgery, when I was discharged. My drains were still attached and my husband insisted on taking me to a movie instead of taking me home (where I wanted to go feel sad for myself and mourn my loss). I don't even remember the movie but from that moment on it did set the pace for how we would deal with this life "interruption."

When You Get Home: Post-Mastectomy or Lumpectomy

Wear nursing pads on your boobies with loose tank tops. Don't look at the dust bunnies.

☐ Schedule friends/family to bathe you. It's weird, I know, but you really will need some help.

☐ Have someone with you 24/7 for at least 7-10 days after you get home.

☐ Have someone open all containers at home—pill bottles, jelly jars, etc. You won't have the strength in your hands to open anything after surgery.

☐ Have someone place everything you need at elbow height, be it on your bedroom or bathroom shelf. You can't reach up.

☐ You need people to drive you around for at least several weeks. Ask your doctor for the length of time needed.

I'll say it again and again: *learn to receive!* It is not easy for us women who are natural givers. This is the time to receive and to allow yourself to be pampered. It can be a beautiful thing. Really!

Laugh! Watch funny videos.

Focus on you. Not work. Not others. YOU. YOU. YOU. Be selfish. It's okay. And healthy. And healing.

Visiting Nurse and Drains

I mentioned it before, but in case you forgot to do this, have your doctor order a visiting nurse to come to your home every day to clean the drains. If insurance will pay for that, get it. It can't hurt and it will help. It also puts less stress on those around you to help you with the drains.

Removal of Drains

Before going to get your drains removed, take strong pain medicines. Ask your doctor first, of course.

Physical Therapy and Lymphedema

Within the first four weeks after surgery, go to a physical therapist who is certified specifically in lymphedema so they can guide you in the proper direction in performing range of motion activities and exercises in an effort to keep moving and stay strong. Also get in a habit of comparing your arms. After surgery it is normal for the affected side to be swollen over the quadrant. Occasionally the arm will stay this way until you start moving it and regain your range of motion and strength as mentioned. Now if the affected arm or quadrant does not decrease in swelling within a month, have it reassessed by your doctor or therapist.

Here are a few lymphedema symptoms that you can be on the lookout for:
• Swelling of the fingers and arm
• Sores in the skin
• Fitted clothing not easy to wear
• Your arm feels tight (full)
• It's not easy to move your affected joints
• Your shoulder is sore due to your arm having increased weight
• Your old rings, bracelets, or watches are tight

These precautions apply to the arm/upper trunk area on the side of the surgery only:

- No heavy lifting until you control the swelling (remember to talk to your lymphedema/physical therapist.)
- No withdrawal of blood from that arm. Ever.
- No blood pressure checks on that arm. Ever.
- Avoid cuts and insect bites. (If you do sustain one, use an antibacterial topical cream such as Neosporin® and observe it. If it doesn't heal or looks worse, go to your doctor for follow-up.)
- Use an electric shaver for underarm. NO razors!
- No cutting of cuticles with manicures.
- Use your compression garment (sleeve) while exercising and/or when traveling in a plane.
- Maintain your ideal body weight.
- Exercise. Ask your physical therapist to guide you in an appropriate program for you.
- Don't wear anything with tight sleeves, cuffs, or tight jewelry.
- Move: Don't sit in any one spot for more than 20 minutes.
- As much as possible, keep your arm positioned above your heart for periods at a time.
- Carry your purse on the opposite shoulder.
- Do not use a heating pad on the affected arm.

Scarring

Ask your plastic surgeon what you should do for scarring. Some have recommended:

- Vitamin E oil for minimizing scarring. But ask your doctor first just to be sure it's okay.
- Kelo-cote® (advanced formula scar gel for $40 at your local pharmacy).

Radiation: Energy Zapper

I didn't have radiation, but many women do. Here are tips from several Sistas who did:

- If you can have someone go with you to the appointments, do it. It does not have to be every time or the same person, but having company makes it more enjoyable. The appointments are usually pretty brief, but they are daily. The novelty wears off.

- Make sure you ask about special parking rates for daily appointment-goers. If you have a distance to travel for appointments or your hospital is in a major city, plan to visit the local museum before or after an appointment or treat yourself to a nice meal.

- Talk to the others who seem friendly in the waiting area. They are all in the same boat and it is nice to make a new friend.

- You will have a procedure they call "mapping." This involves a CT scan of your chest area.

They want to see where everything inside is and how the radiation beam will travel in your body. If you will be radiated on the left side, they want to make sure the radiation does not impact your heart. Some doctors will ask you to do a breath hold. This way they can compare where your heart and lungs are positioned with and without a breath hold. Not every radiation oncologist uses breath holds. Ask if they do use it and if not, why?

• A team will review all of the films of your chest area to make the plan. Remember, this is the plan for your body. You can ask to see the films and have them explain the dosing of the radiation and show you how it will travel through your body. It makes more sense with pictures.

• Guided imagery while they are radiating you can be very helpful. I learned mine from **Removing the Dross** by Nancy Hopps. I also liked the selection of guided imagery available from the website **www.healthjourneys.com**.

• I named the radiation machine "Friend" and I thanked it for its accuracy and precision in delivering the radiant healing light at each session. After a while, I even saw a kind of smiley face in the "face" of the machine.

• Buy men's cotton t-shirts to wear as your new 'bras.' The area will be very tender.

• Hydrate your skin three times a day with Crème moisturizer.

• When the skin gets dark, put on hydrocortisone one percent cream and then Elta (super emollient cream).

• To relieve burn or redness, use fresh aloe from an aloe plant. Keep it in the refrigerator. It's healing, cold, and feels so good. Wrap unused aloe plant in paper towel and keep refrigerated. This did more for some than any cream or lotion.

• Start moisturizing your chest area as soon as the surgeon says it is okay to do so. Check with the radiation oncologist or the radiation nurse on which is the best product to use. Ask for the manufacturer's email address to send the list of ingredients of moisturizers to help you make the best choice. I used Aquaphor®. The radiation dries your skin so getting a head start on moisturizing helps. Hydrate, hydrate, hydrate! Moisturize and drink a lot of water. I brought my moisturizer with me and reapplied immediately following the session.

• Save some old t-shirts to put on right after applying the moisturizer, especially if using something as oily as Aquaphor. The shirts will likely get stained.

• If your skin gets burned and dark, clean it twice a day with Domeboro®. You can purchase it at your local pharmacy.
  – Have someone help you with this process. When mixing it with water have them put on a mask to avoid inhaling it.
  – Have a white cotton hand towel and soak it in distilled water and place it on the radiated skin.
  – It refreshes the skin and feels so soothing.

— Ask your doctor to write a prescription for silver sulfadiazine. It is a white cream that heals skin infections. A friend of mine that is a nurse refers to this as "skin Clorox®."

— Cover the radiated skin with the silver sulfadiazine before you go to sleep. You will see and feel the difference and how it will soothe the skin burn.

- Get plenty of rest. Your body is busy healing even if the skin still looks good. Everyone's skin reacts differently. Talk to your doctor or nurse about any changes to your skin or experiences of pain.

- Focus on gratitude!

- As always, check with your doctor on all of the above!

 Oncologist Visit

Prepare for your visit to the oncologist the same way you prepared for your visit to the surgeon. Get your list of questions from websites such as the American Cancer Society's website. **www.cancer.org.**

Questions would include:

☐ What treatment choices do I have?

☐ Which treatment do you recommend, and why?

☐ What are the risks and side effects of the treatments you recommend?

☐ What should I do to be ready for treatment?

☐ How long will treatment last? What will it involve? Where will it be done?

☐ How will treatment affect my daily activities?

A Sista wrote:

"Make sure to ask lots of questions. You can even ask to record the session if you have a little handheld device. Some doctors are a bit reluctant, but stand your ground and they usually agree. I joked with them about a terrible memory and my husband not remembering things to my preferred level of detail. I found it was too hard to take notes for both of us. We were too emotionally invested. I liked listening to the recordings after the appointment. It generated more questions after listening or I had questions answered by listening again. It takes a while for some information to sink in or to even make sense."

Really spend time with your doctor and his or her head nurse or office manager. Work with them as far as your insurance goes. What is covered and what isn't? Educate yourself so you're not surprised at the end of the day.

If chemo is your treatment, ask your oncologist:

☐ About the chemo drugs and why they are needed. Get all the information you can.

☐ For a prescription in case you get an upset stomach during chemo.

☐ For a prescription for sleep medication. DXM was one of my pre-meds and it made me wired. Ask your doctor.

☐ About Neulasta®. It is a magic shot that helps boost your immune system after chemo. Ask your oncologist about it. Here's a link for more information: **www.neulasta.com**. You normally get it 24 hours after chemo. It helps to get it in the belly, where there's fat. I thought it would be painful, but I really didn't feel it there.

☐ To order your blood work a day or two before chemo and not the "day of." Otherwise you'll spend even more hours in the hospital as you wait for the results before chemo can start.

☐ What you *can* and *cannot* eat.

☐ For an appointment with the hospital nutritionist.

☐ What supplements you can take while undergoing chemo. Mine told me I could only take two supplements:

   – At least 500 mg of calcium/day (more if recommended for you)
   – Vitamin D

☐ For a lidocaine prescription. It's a numbing cream (sometimes called EMLA Cream®.) Spread the cream on the port area one hour before going to chemo. The cream will numb your skin so you don't feel chemo IV needle going in. Once you put the cream on, cover it with Saran™ wrap so your clothing doesn't wipe it off. Put this in your calendar as a recurring appointment before each chemo treatment or for days when you have blood drawn.

☐ About acupuncture during chemo. Many patients swear by it. Ask your doctor what he/she thinks. If it's recommended, your insurance company might cover it and some hospitals offer it.

☐ If psychological counseling is necessary and ask for a recommendation.

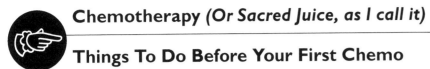

Chemotherapy (Or Sacred Juice, as I call it)

Things To Do Before Your First Chemo

Wig shopping

Make shopping for wigs fun. Do it before you start to lose your hair.

☐ Synthetic wigs are easier to care for; they already come with a do.

☐ Check with your insurance company. Many cover it. It is called a cranial prosthesis.

☐ We found two companies you might want to check out:

- www.PaulaYoung.com: cost efficient wigs
- www.headcovers.com: soft hats that keep your head warm

Cut your hair

☐ Do this before chemo starts or after your first chemo. It will make the transition to baldness easier, if you it short now.

Organize your pills

☐ Organize your pill bottles before each chemo treatment. I had Zantac®, (to prevent heartburn) that I took the day before chemo, morning and night; DMX (short for dexamethasone, to prevent nausea and vomiting) that I took the day before, the day of and the day after chemo; and Emend (three pills for nausea the day before, day of and day after.) It's confusing, especially with chemo brain and fatigue. Sign up a friend to help you organize the meds. It can be overwhelming. Once again, place a pill reminder in your calendar as a recurring appointment before each chemo treatment.

Grooming and Beauty

☐ Get a manicure and pedicure. You can't have them during treatment due to a risk of infection.

☐ Dye your gray hairs. You can't do that during treatment either.

☐ Get long hair cut as short as you can stand before it starts to fall out. It won't be as traumatic that way when it falls out. And then when it does start to fall out, shave it right away. I waited too long. Believe it or not, you'll look cool bald.

Preparing Your Home and Pets For Life During Chemo

Have an angel come and clean your home the day before every chemo treatment. Here's a great idea: Download an application from this website: **www.cleaningforareason.org**—and have it signed by your doctor. They will send someone to do basic cleaning of your home, free of charge, during chemo treatment. This will occur once per month during four months. This organization serves the entire USA and currently has 547 partners to help these women.

• If you have cats, stay away from the litter box. Germs and more germs. I had a friend, a true friend (Annie) clean my litter box every single day for one year. Find your own angel.

 You can't be around animals that aren't yours. It's okay to be around those that your body recognizes, but you can't be around others until after you're done with chemo.

• Also, to avoid germs, some friends I know use white linens on the sofa on a daily basis and wash them in Clorox® along with the towels. It keeps everything clean. However, some cannot stand the smell of Clorox during treatment. Listen to your body!

The Day Before Every Chemo and Blood Test

If you have tiny veins like I do and you don't have a port, here are a few tips to juice up your veins:

• Drink tons of fluid the day before. Especially Gatorade®.

• Eat Chinese food the night before. This will give you lots of sodium.

• Wear long sleeves to keep your arms warm. Veins shrivel up if they're cold.

• When you arrive to have blood drawn, ask for a heating pad to heat your veins.

• Ask for a butterfly needle. Finding veins is usually easier with one. A butterfly needle is a short needle with a small diameter attached to a thin, flexible tube.

Heading to Chemo

I started each chemo session day with a little prayer and meditation before leaving my house.

Bring whatever is sacred and comforting to you. These are things I brought to each chemo treatment:

• An angel or two. It makes the day go by faster and it's fun to have angels with you

- My "mesa." It's a little bag filled with my sacred stones

- Soothing Native American flute music

- Camera to document the journey

- Hand fan

- Snacks

- Journal

Remember to spread the lidocaine cream over your port area, cover it with Saran Wrap and put a little jacket over it. You won't feel a thing after that. I never felt the chemo needle go in. I LOVE lidocaine!

I took a "breath" before every treatment by either going to my yard or stopping somewhere in nature on the way to the hospital. Sometimes I just went to my corner bakery with my angels. This will help calm you down so you can be more relaxed and at peace when you get there.

When you arrive at the hospital, signing in takes a while. Then they'll search for the blood results. You'll be weighed in and asked a bunch of questions.

Be patient! Be kind and loving to everyone there. They're your healers!

Once you're in the system, then you'll be taken to a cubicle where you will meet your wonderful chemo nurse. These people are sent from above. You'll wait a while for the official doctor's order to start chemo. Sometimes for a long while. They need to know your blood results and weight that day to know exactly how much chemo to give you. It's a process. BE PATIENT.

Let me talk about patience again. Patience is key here. When you're going through chemo, it's going to take a while. It's a long process. The waiting room is full of people. If you come knowing that, it's okay. Bring a book. Bring a friend. Bring happiness and joy. Bring patience!

As the chemo goes into your system, accept it, love it, welcome it. Visualize it doing great things in your body. Manifest healing. You are more powerful than you think. Then express gratitude that you're alive at a time when Sacred Juice exists and you have access to it!

As soon as the chemo goes into your body, it needs to come out. Hydrate yourself. Drink lots of water while they infuse you and afterwards when you go home.

Have fun with your chemo nurses. They work very hard every day. They'd appreciate humor and fun.

Dancing Your Way Through Chemo (I call it the *Chemo Conga*)

Four basic chemo tips:

1. Drink lots of water.

2. The 8-10 days after your chemo treatment is called NADIR. The word NADIR comes from Old French and Arabic terms. It means "the lowest point." This refers to the blood counts, particularly white blood cell count and platelet count. NADIR refers to when your immune system is most suppressed. That's when you really, really need to be careful not to catch anything from anyone. I avoided crowds during that time like the plague!

3. Keep yourself and your home sanitized. Use hand sanitizer products (my doctors always recommended Dial® anti-bacterial soap.) Use it often and have bottles throughout the house. Wash your hands a LOT. You and everyone who comes near you should wash their hands. Don't be shy. It's your health!

4. Limit hugging and kissing. Of course we all need loving, especially at a time like this. But we don't want the germs.

Chemo Cuisine

The Basics

Everyone is different. These are the things that worked for me and/or for friends who went through chemo. But listen to your own body. Ask your doctor before doing anything. I always made a list of things I wanted to eat/drink and would run it by my oncologist. As far as food goes, ask your doctor to order an appointment with your hospital nutritionist and make sure that your insurance company will pay for it.

- Before each meal, I was told to drink 8-16 ounces of water. Sometimes I could do that, other times I just couldn't.

- 5-10 minutes of breath work (yoga if possible) before each meal.

- WASH your mouth with warm water and baking soda AFTER every single meal. This kills bacteria in your mouth.

When you undergo cancer treatment, you can develop a weakened immune system. Avoiding food-borne illnesses is essential. To help prevent food borne illnesses:

- Wash all fruits and vegetables thoroughly with a veggie scrubbing pad, even if you plan on peeling the fruit or vegetable. Tammi, Lydia, and Annie used to even scrub my strawberries one by one. So sweet!

- Buy a veggie wash. They're sold at most supermarkets. A friend recommended a do-it-yourself wash: one part hydrogen peroxide to 10 parts water. I never tried this and if you do, ask your doctor first!

- Wash your hands and food preparation surfaces before and after preparing food, especially after handling raw meat.

- Thaw meat in the refrigerator, not on the kitchen counter.

- Avoid raw shellfish and sushi.

- Pre-packaged salad mixes are *NOT* germ-free. Triple-washed may still have pathogens lurking in the greens, so wash them before eating.

Easy Way To Calculate Healthy Meals

Starch	1 fist
Fruit	1 fist
Milk	1 fist
Vegetables, non-starchy	2 fists
Very lean meat, poultry, low-fat cottage cheese, egg beaters	1 palm
Fat, oils, nuts, avocado:	1 thumb

 ## Dos and Don'ts

Do:
- Have DISTILLED water or boiled water if possible.

- Eat as much as you can because you don't want to lose weight. Your body needs that fuel and energy to keep moving. Don't worry about dieting now. So even if you have to eat 10 to 12 times a day, do it.

- Your taste for food might change with every chemo. Buy some basics before, but maybe consider what my friend Muriel did:
  "I never bought groceries beforehand. I would go after chemo and do the "looksy diet." Whatever I saw that looked appealing, I would buy it. Of course, I tried to be healthy in my choices, too."

- Buy popsicles. Sometimes they're really soothing.

- Have something to eat the nanosecond you open your eyes. I had to, otherwise I would get nauseous. So I always had something next to my bed—nuts or breads—something to pop into my mouth the moment I woke up in the morning.

- Drink plenty of liquids between meals, at least 1 hour before and 1 hour after meals.

- Drink ginger ale, ginger tea, and peppermint tea. They have anti-nausea/stomach settling properties.

- Include sea-salted vegetable broths or miso broth in your diet if you are experiencing vomiting and severe diarrhea. These salty additions will help to keep your electrolytes balanced and can revive you when you are feeling faint. (Miso is a salty paste made from soybeans and can be found in health food stores, Asian food markets and some supermarkets.)

- Eat smaller, more frequent meals. Five or six snack-type meals a day can reduce some of the stress on your digestive tract. Smoothies make a perfect meal.

- Include vegetables and fruit juices (fresh squeezed for the highest nutrient content, if possible) and clear broths. BUT wash everything beforehand.

- Use only pasteurized or processed ciders and juices and pasteurized milk and cheese.

- Drink ½ aloe vera juice, ½ apple juice in the morning before breakfast.

- Have a protein drink in the morning with banana. Whole wheat toast with almond butter, which is better than peanut butter.

- Eat a well-balanced diet. ***Lots of protein is the key to chemo!*** Protein is important for white blood cells to go up. Eggs, chicken, beans, and nuts (almonds and walnuts, particularly).

- Be sure to cook meat and eggs thoroughly. Make sure the carton says they're pasteurized and never buy a dozen that contains any obvious cracks or leaks.

- Eat lots of fruits and vegetables (especially dark leafy green ones) for different vitamins, minerals and antioxidants that the body WILL need to repair. I also found red and orange vegetables are great immune-boosters. You will get these via the natural way which will not interfere with chemo. *But wash and cook everything*!

- Eat healthy carbs. Main calories will come from carbs in whole grain. For example, eat whole wheat bread, brown rice, whole wheat pasta, and starchy vegetables (potatoes and sweet potatoes). Sweet potatoes are high in antioxidants. Carbs will keep the energy levels up.

- If you're going to eat meat, then eat lean meats. Take off skin. Eat lean beef, organic chicken, and turkey (NO PORK).

- Have olive oil and almond butter in moderation. They have good fat. Two tablespoons of almond butter has the same amount of protein as an egg. An ounce or two of cheese will equal the protein in one egg.

- Eat low-fat rather than normal cheese.

- Indulge in beans. They are a great source of protein.

- Enjoy your fish. They contain Omega-3 fatty acids and are a high source of protein. Mix them up. Don't eat the same fish all the time. Omega-3 is found in fish such as salmon, tuna, and halibut, other seafood including algae and krill, some plants, and nut oils. They are anti-inflammatory.

- One of the things that worked for me was to eat those little Argentinean sandwiches you can buy at Argentine restaurants.

- Spice up your food with garlic, if your stomach can take it. It's great for the immune system.

- Enjoy your mushrooms, cooked and washed really, really well. Shitake mushrooms are full of lentinan, an anti-tumor enzyme.

- And last, but certainly not least, **GO ORGANIC**! They will eliminate exposure to chemicals and pesticides.

Clean 15: Lowest in Pesticides	Dirty Dozen: Worst in Pesticides
Avocado	Peach
Onion	Apple
Sweet Corn	Bell Pepper
Pineapple	Celery
Mango	Nectarine
Asparagus	Strawberries
Sweet Peas	Cherries
Kiwi	Kale
Cabbage	Lettuce
Eggplant	Grapes (imported)
Papaya	Carrot
Watermelon	Pear
Broccoli	
Tomato	
Sweet Potato	

See full list at **www.foodnews.org**

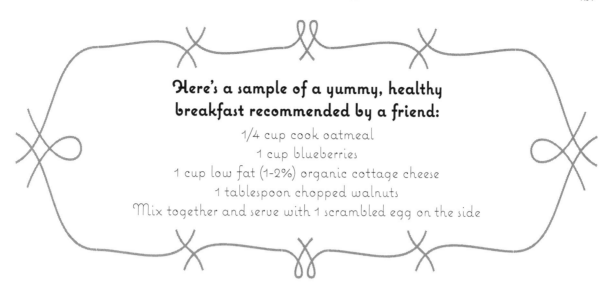

Here's a sample of a yummy, healthy breakfast recommended by a friend:

1/4 cup cook oatmeal
1 cup blueberries
1 cup low fat (1-2%) organic cottage cheese
1 tablespoon chopped walnuts
Mix together and serve with 1 scrambled egg on the side

Don'ts:

- No drinking of **herbal** or **green** teas during chemo treatment. Some studies have indicated that some herbal, green, and black tea extracts stimulate genes that cause cells to be less sensitive to chemotherapy drugs. Given this potential interaction, people should not drink black, green, and some herbal teas (as well as extracts of these teas) while receiving chemotherapy. Ask your doctor.

- No eating of leftovers of any food older than 24 hours.

- Don't lie down after eating. Allow yourself an hour or more to digest.

- Do not drink liquids WITH your meals. This keeps your digestive juices at full strength, promoting complete digestion and reducing indigestion.

- Stay away from sugar as it can increase your risk for intestinal Candida infection that is very common at this vulnerable time. If you must use a sweetener, use a grain-derived sweetener like rice syrup or barley malt.

- Some steroids (which are part of chemo premeds) can make your blood sugar elevated. If blood sugar is elevated, it will be a source for the cancer cells to grow. Sugar and desserts are NOT GOOD. As my oncologist said to me "Sugar is cancer's best friend."

- Avoid all fatty foods. Focus your diet on fresh fruits, steamed or boiled vegetables, light grains, and proteins.

- Don't overdo fats. Unsaturated fats are okay, with one teaspoon per meal.

- Don't eat fried foods and don't cook with sauces and gravies.

- Avoid the "bad" fats. Saturated fats come mostly from animals and raise the level of cholesterol in your blood.

- Do not have honey if it is not pasteurized. You can cook with the honey since it will be heated.

- Stay away from restaurants during chemo. MOST patients that end up in the hospital during chemo with a fever have eaten at a restaurant. Exposure to bacteria is high at restaurants since you don't know how they handle the food. Dairy products may be kept out too long and hand washing may not be optimal.

- Stay away from organ meats (such as liver steak.) They are not good since the liver filters all pesticides and bacteria. The organ meats are also very high in cholesterol.

- Don't take fish oil or flaxseed oil supplements. Fish oils from eating fish are fine but don't take pills during chemo since it is not known if it interferes with chemo.

- Stay away from processed foods and foods that are not natural (like fake sugar) because the body has no idea what to do with them.

Metallic Taste and Mouth Sores

I experienced a metallic taste when undergoing chemo. Many people do. This taste can alter the way food tastes and at times you smell burning metal over and over again. It's very weird.

Some tips to alleviate this:
- Use mint in your food.
- Suck on mints and lemon drop candy.
- Ask your doctor for a prescription for a white milky liquid that really helps alleviate this as well as the mouth sores which you might get.
- Some good dill pickles. No kidding.
- Eat with plastic utensils instead of silver or metal ones.

Hair Today, Bald Tomorrow

You are NOT your hair. You aren't even your breasts. But getting back to you hair. Yes, you will be bald. Big deal. It grows back. Of course, I went through my own emotional roller coaster, but eventually I snapped out of it. Now I love my new hair even more than my original hair.

Dealing With Hair Loss
- Shave as soon as you can. I waited too long. Now looking back at pictures I see how "sick" I looked with wisps of hair. On the other hand, I looked pretty cool bald. So shave!

- For me a satin pillow case was a life-saver. The skin on my head hurt a LOT when I lost my hair. It was painful to lay my head on a pillow. So a friend recommended and bought a satin pillow case for me. It was magical. No more pain. Like I keep saying, everyone is different. For another friend, 100 percent cotton helped her more than the satin. Do what works for you.

• Have fun with the hats, wigs, and bandanas you bought. Be someone new every day!

• After treatment ends and you're bald, massage Rosemary Hair Oil on your scalp. The benefits are:

    – Stimulating follicles which results in longer and stronger hair.

    – Boosting mental activity. Rosemary oil is an excellent brain and nerve tonic and a good remedy for depression, mental fatigue, and forgetfulness. Inhaling rosemary oil lifts your spirits immediately. Whenever your brain is tired, inhale rosemary oil to remove boredom and get fresh mental energy. It is not only soothing, but feels feminine as well.

 Exercise

I used chemo as an excuse not to exercise and this was a huge mistake. The opposite is what's recommended.

Try a short walk after meals or, if you need to rest, sit with your legs stretched out and your head propped up with pillows.

Stay active. You will do better if your muscles are strong and your metabolism is stimulated. Yoga is the BEST!

 Chemo Brain

Your memory will get fuzzy. You will become forgetful. It's normal and eventually your memory does come back. So don't freak out about it.

• Eat your veggies. Studies have shown that eating more vegetables is linked to keeping brain power as people age.

• Set up and follow routines.

• Pick a certain place for commonly lost objects and put them there each time. Try to keep the same daily schedule.

• Don't try to multi-task. Focus on one thing at a time.

- Ask for help when you need it. Friends and loved ones can help with daily tasks to cut down on distractions and help you save mental energy.

The real issue here is that recovery from cancer treatment is not always a one-year process but can even be a two- to five-year process. People need to understand the extent to which the cells in their bodies have really been compromised by not only the cancer, but also the treatment. One of the things I would complain a lot about during treatment is word finding—you know the word, it's a tip-of-the-tongue experience—but I couldn't come up with it. The happy news is that that piece of cognitive function does recover, but it usually takes longer than a year. I'm going on a year and a half and I have my memory back.

Laugh about it. It gives you an excuse to do silly things!

 ## Dry Skin, Eyes, And Throat

Chemo can dry out your skin. Here are some tips to help:
- Drink lots of fluids especially water prior, during and after chemo. It will help with the dryness the body endures each time.

- Buy a product called Aquaphor®. The hands, feet, and nails get brittle with chemo. Put this on every night.

- Try Eucerin® Dry Skin Therapy - Everyday Protection Body Lotion with SPF 15.

- I loved all the Aveeno® Moisturizers.

- Use Biotene® Mouth Wash to relieve dry mouth.

- Use Biotene® Oral Balance Dry Mouth Moisturizer gel. Spread it over your tongue. It will help with the dryness, specifically after chemo and for days afterwards.

- For dry lips, use Blistex® DCT SPF 20.

- For dry eyes, use Blink Tears®. If you wear contact lenses, use Blink Contacts®.

This tip is from a friend who took Taxotere. I'm putting it here so you can ask your oncologist.
"I have never had allergies and I finally figured out that because Taxotere is made from plant alkaloids, I was just having a good ole' allergic reaction. My throat and nose feel dry. I can drink gallons of water for my throat, but the best thing is to take a lozenge like Halls® or Ricola®. Now for the nose. Vicks® VapoRub (or the CVS/Walgreens generic) works wonders. My nose has felt like sandpaper for the past three days but since I gently applied some VapoRub in both nostrils, it's like my nose is finally saying 'Aahhh, thank you.' It feels much smoother up there."

When Treatment Ends

Celebrate!

- Don't go back to your crazy life. Learn to balance. You don't want a repeat performance.

- Follow up with your post treatment appointments. Because I was on chemo for a year, I developed a bit of osteoporosis and had to go on Fosomax® to build up bone mass loss. Because I was on Herceptin, I continue to see my cardiologist on a regular basis since Herceptin sometimes causes damage to the heart muscle. Stay serious about all follow-up appointments.

- Pay it forward. I can't stress that enough. Take what you've gone through and make a difference in the lives of others.

- Work with support groups, a psychologist or anyone who can help you figure out your new life after cancer. It can be beautiful and joyful in ways you never expected.

- I brought together the Link of Hope Sistas, created Positively Pat, am producing TV shows and writing books such as this one. My mission is to do everything I can to pay it forward.

- My Sista Rhonda Smith is now dedicating herself to help survivors with her website and community. **www.breastcancerpartner.com**

  ### Rhonda states it eloquently:
  "Once surgery, chemotherapy, and radiation treatment are over, there is no manual, prescription or remedy to help you recover from the physical, emotional, and mental impact of the experience, nor help you restore yourself back to normal, whatever that may be.

  "Although you probably have been looking forward to the day when treatment is over, it may seem a bit anticlimactic when you're finally done, and you may find yourself pondering 'What do I do now?'

  "Your medical team is no longer an integral part of your nearly everyday routine, and you're left to your own devices to care for yourself and figure out how to live beyond breast cancer and get your life back on track. Aside from the cycle of periodic check-ups and diagnostic tests, your recovery is all up to you.

  "So, what do you do? Breast Cancer Partner provides answers to this question. It is a resource for developing your roadmap to recovery—a plan to help you navigate your way through the healing process. We encourage you to take advantage of the resources and information provided to help you make the appropriate choices in managing your overall health and well-being so that your recovery occurs with ease and is as successful as possible."

- Cindy Papale wrote the book, **The Empty Cup Runneth Over,** to help breast cancer patients and is now working on a movie. **www.theemptycuprunnethover.com**

- Carolyn Newman, another Sista, is all about educating women on lymphedema. She has to wear a sleeve 24/7 and didn't feel very pretty in it. So she actually started her own company, Warrior Wear. She created *Arm Candy,* which is a decorative outer sleeve that is designed to provide a more fashionable look for those who have to wear compression arm sleeves. It also protects your compression garment without adding extra compression! **www.warriorwear4u.com**

- Other Link of Hope Sistas are paying it forward in their own way. You'll meet them on **www.PositivelyPat.com**.

- Don't stress. Live in the now; that's all any of us really have. Be happy.

- Oh, and of course, don't sweat the small stuff. *Enjoy your life!* It's a beautiful thing.

You've been given the gift of life. Honor it. Celebrate every day as your Re-Birthday! Live in gratitude.

Epilogue

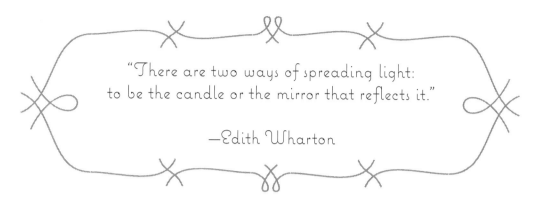

"There are two ways of spreading light:
to be the candle or the mirror that reflects it."

—Edith Wharton

Life is different now. In a good way.

The most challenging part for me is not falling back into the old patterns of working and rushing and doing and being in a constant state of motion. It tries to creep up on me on most days, but either I notice or those around me do.

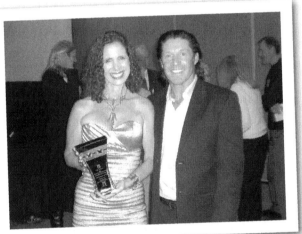

I still run San Pedro Productions, my public relations and marketing production company. I was honored earlier this year with the Coral Gables Chamber Business **Woman of the Year Award** in Philanthropy.

I am also working on a variety of projects that have become my mission and passion.

Business Woman of the Year with Patricio

1. Facilitating a community of breast cancer patients, survivors, and their caregivers, called **Positively Pat**. It's grown to be a home where some pretty cool people, such as the **Link of Hope Sistas,** along with experts in their fields, share health and wellness tips, information, important medical breakthroughs, and spiritual insights. **www.PositivelyPat.com** is a portal of information with a community that reaches across the globe from Ireland to North Carolina; from England to Paris; from Italy to Argentina; and from Atlanta to Miami. There are no borders for this community of hope and healing. I hope you'll visit often and let your friends and family know about us.

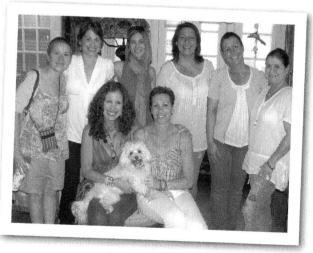

Link of Hope Sistas 2011

2. My healing journey is about to air on ***Discovery Home & Health,*** and on ***Discovery Familia.*** It is a one-hour documentary that I am co-producing with them and Imagina U.S. The special will air in October 2011 in Latin American and US Hispanic markets. It's called ***Why NOT Me*** (Tengo Cáncer) and it's the realization of the vision that I had the night before I was diagnosed with breast cancer. My goal is to take this documentary around the world to impact as many people as possible.

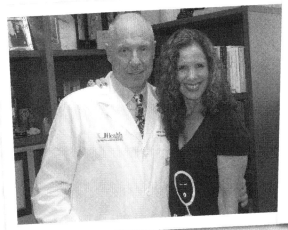 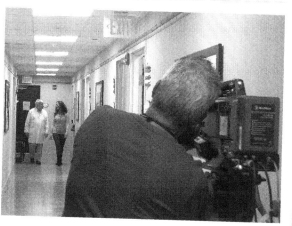

I interviewed Dr. Glück for my Discovery special   *Dr. D provided great info for documentary*

3. Photography has always been a passion for me. I drive my friends crazy because I never go anywhere without my camera in hand, especially during my breast cancer journey. Now that passion is becoming a reality as I am exhibiting **Discover Your Doorway** at galleries across the country. This is a 3-D, interactive, mixed-media exhibit that incorporates woodwork and photos of beautiful doors, that when opened, reveal breathtaking landscapes.

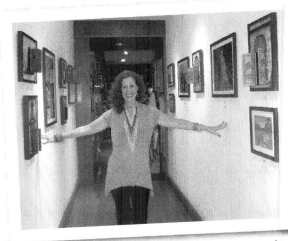 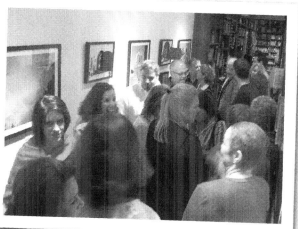

Discover Your Doorway. My first photo exhibit   *A packed opening night*

4. Then there is this book. I've been writing it for three years with the help of angels. I believe that when you're on the right path, everything will flow smoothly. Since the moment I made the decision to use my breast cancer experience to help others, I've been led on the path. I've trusted that everything was happening exactly as it needed to and that time would unveil what I had to do.

After going through two years of chemo-brain, where I could hardly concentrate or focus on the simplest of tasks, I am now multi-tasking many projects with many legs. Yet I'm doing it from a place of peace. You would think that I would be overwhelmed. But I'm not. Angels fell from the heavens into my lap.

Acknowledgements

Co-Writer
Tammi Leader Fuller (Miami, Florida and now Los Angeles, California)

I put out a call for help through *LinkedIn* and the call was answered. These are my angels who are working with me on all my projects—pro bono. They all have a drive, a purpose and a mission to be of service. I love each and every one of them although I've never met some of them in person. It doesn't just take a community, it takes a planet of compassion, care and love. Thank you.

Book Editor
Lorraine Fico-White • www.magnificomanuscripts.com (Charlotte, North Carolina)
You are a true professional. But your humanity is what touched my heart. Thank you for editing this book with such warmth, compassion, and humor. You are a joy to work with.

Contributing Editors
Loren Kleinman • www.lkeditorial.com (Montclair, New Jersey)
Kristen "Kitty" Collins • collinsk711@gmail.com (St. Louis, Missouri)
Pat Naegle • patnaegle@gmail.com (Tampa, Florida)

Tip Editors
Debbie Cabrera • (Miami, Florida)
Sue Hampton-Mathews • sueh_m@hotmail.com (United Kingdom)
Marlena Wood (Miami, Florida)

Graphic Designer/Art Director/Proofer
Shannon E. Coffey • secoffey@bellsouth.net • www.behance.net/artifactstudio
(Atlanta, Georgia)
Your passion, creativity, professionalism and attention to detail are amazing. You've taken this project on with the force of a tornado. You're a gem to work with and I'm so grateful for all you're doing. THANK YOU.

eBook Publishing Designer
Kevin O. McLaughlin • www.kevinomclaughlin.com (Burlington, Vermont)

Cover Phototographer
Mark Dietz

Content Providers
Gilda Alonso
Sally Bogert
Maria Bradman
Paula Holland De Long
Claudia Edwards
Cecilia Fernandez Hall
Judy Hurley
Link of Hope Sistas

Teresita Machado
Patricio Madariaga
Ana Mendieta
Carolyn Newman
Randi Leader Oakes
Lydia Sacasa
Annie San Roman
Muriel Sommers
Pilar Uribe

Speechwriter
Sonny Catalano

My Healers
All my angels
All the nurses and nurse assistants at:
- UM Sylvester Comprehensive Cancer
- Baptist Outpatient Services
- Baptist Health Systems
- Breast Diagnostics

Dr. Vilma Biaggi
Dr. Robert DerHagopian
Dr. Claudia Edwards
Dr. Stefan Glück
Rev. Chris Jackson
Haydee Kapin
Brian Keely
Jacqui Kelly LMT
Rev. Elizabeth Longo
Dr. Dierdre Marshall
Orfirio "Max" Sanchez (RN)
Christian Leon Otrakji, MD, Associate Pathologist
Emilio Solares PT
Dr. Myles Starkman DC
Unity on the Bay
Dr. Alberto Villoldo
Hadi Yaziji MD

My Web Guru
Jayme Lam • www.4thReaction.com (Miami, Florida)
I can't thank you enough for all you're done for me over the years. You brought *Positively Pat* to life in 2008 with a beautiful website. I'm so grateful to you for your continued love and support. Your kindness and creativity have taken *Positively Pat* to new heights. Thank you for wanting to make a difference. Thank you for the hours spent on bringing the new site and vision to life.

Web Assistance
Kevin Ference (Jacksonville, Florida)

Social Media Strategist
Fernando Fonseca • www.thezargon.org (Seattle, Washington)
Thank you for giving of yourself and helping me spread my wings across social media.

Social Media Assistants
Debbie Cabrera
Lori Davis
Vicky Marquez
Angelica Melo • www.afterdarknetwork.co.uk (UK)

www.PositivelyPat.com Editor
Terry Aguayo • AGUAYOT@aol.com (Miami, Florida)
Thank you for your willingness to help edit my website when I still wasn't able to fully focus.

IT
Robert Sante (Miami, Florida)
Thank you for always coming through for me when I hit the panic button on my computer!

My Lawyer
Alan Rosenthal (Miami, Florida)
Thank you for always being willing to help, and for keeping me legal.

Video Editors/Photographers
Lori Davis (Miami, Florida)
You always go above and beyond to be of service. From editing my videos to doing whatever is needed. No matter what. Thank you for the love and countless hours of work you've donated to this project. You are a true friend.

Dale West (dale@dalewestvideo.tv), Jaime Quintana (5iveyearplan@gmail.com), and Chris Nickless (Miami, Florida)

Thank you for ALL the editing and shooting you both did. You were always there for me, no matter how last minute. You were supportive, compassionate, and kind and I will forever be grateful.

Still Photographer
George Butch (Plantation, Florida)
Thank you for your kindness in doing my photo shoots so I could document the phases of my hair.

Translators/Editors
This book (and www.PositivelyPat.com) will travel the world. These are the translators who are making it possible:

Spanish
- Cristina Heraud de van Tol • www.vantol-heraud.com (Peru)
- Adela Morales • adelasmorales@aol.com (Miami, Florida)
- Karina Pelech • kapelech@gmail.com (Argentina)
- Jeff and Elvira Burnham • jburnham28@yahoo.com (Indianapolis, Indiana)

Portuguese
- Luana Cavalcanti • www.portuguesetalk.com • luana@portuguesetalk.com (Ireland)
- Rachel Kopit Cunha • Ophicina de Arte & Prosa (Brazil)
- Jonas Nicotra, MEd • jonasnicotra@yahoo.com (Everett, Washington)
- Natalia Sarmiento • www.nataliatraductions.com (Portugal)
- João Nicolau • http://linkedin.com/in/joaon (Portugal)

Italian
- Lucia DiRocco (Italy)

French
- Catherine Zouaoui (France)

Discovery Channel in Miami
Henry Martinez
You believed in my story idea three years ago and now, because of you, it's becoming a Discovery documentary. Thank you!

Books & Books in Miami
Mitchell Kaplan
Cristina Nosti
Thank you for believing in me and supporting all the projects I dream up. You're true friends.

To All The People I Drove Crazy When Trying To Find a Name For This Book
You all know who you are… but special thanks go out to:
Jeanette Hopkins
Carolyn Newman
Both came up with *"Cancer Dancer!"* Thank you.

Plus:
Gemma Cunningham
Tammi Leader Fuller
Kathi and Alan Glist
Link of Hope Sistas
Ritchie Lucas
Patricio Madariaga
Carol and Gary Rosenberg
Lorraine Fico-White
All the Breast Cancer Forums on *LinkedIn*

My Healing Journey Angels
Scott Alan
Jade Alexander
Gilda Alonso
American Airlines Friends
Raymond Bera
Nick Bogert

Sally Bogert
Kathy Bossong (RIP)
Maria Bradman
Camp Bombshell campers
Ivon Carrillo
Lori Davis
Mark Dietz
Will Edwards
Karl and Sylvia Ellins
Stefanie Fallois
Tammi Leader Fuller
Kathi and Alan Glist
Alex and Karina Gonzalez
Tia Marta Gonzalez
Tio Mario Gonzalez
Liza Gross
Barbara Gutierrez
Sandra Haedo
Jeanette Hopkins
Judy Hurley
Joan Leader
Jodi Leader-Allen
Laura Lowe
Charles "Chip" Lunsford
Teresita Machado
Patricio Madariaga
Adela Morales
Randi Leader Oakes
Marcello Rosen (RIP)
Vicky Rua
Lydia Sacasa
Antonio San Pedro
Annie San Roman
Dr. Erika Schwartz
Mercedes Soler
Beverly Stiegler
Rosa Sugrañes
Anne Sussman
Teresita Valdez
Carlos Vallabriga
Bibi Vega
Vivian Wever

You all carried me on your wings to healing. I love you and am grateful for the unconditional and constant support, love, and compassion you blessed me with. I am humbled and filled with love and appreciation. If I left anyone out, I am truly sorry. You still get my forever gratitude.

My Babies
Chloe
Merlot
Pucci
Tango
And my newest addition, Frankie
Thank you for showering me with cuddles and snuggles and healing love.

See you on www.PositivelyPat.com

Notes

Notes

Notes

Notes

Made in the USA
Charleston, SC
10 June 2013